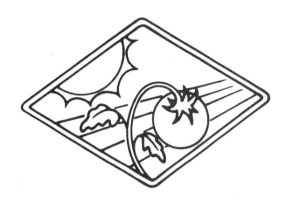

Growing Food

Pamela A. Koch
Angela Calabrese Barton
Isobel R. Contento

**Published by Teachers College Columbia University
and National Gardening Association**

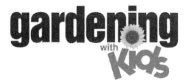

www.KidsGardening.org
www.GardeningWithKids.org

LINKING FOOD AND THE ENVIRONMENT

AN INQUIRY-BASED SCIENCE AND NUTRITION PROGRAM

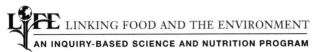

LINKING FOOD AND THE ENVIRONMENT

AN INQUIRY-BASED SCIENCE AND NUTRITION PROGRAM

Linking Food and the Environment (LiFE) is a collaboration of the Science Education and Nutrition Education programs at Teachers College Columbia University established in 1996 with the vision of promoting scientific habits of mind through thoughtful, inquiry-based activities that integrate the study of food, food systems, and environmental and personal health. *Growing Food* is one module of the LiFE Curriculum Series. The mission of all the LiFE modules is to increase scientific conceptual understandings in life science; improve attitudes toward science; improve attitudes toward personal health and nature; and promote behavior changes in relation to personal and ecological health. For information about LiFE, please visit *www.tc.edu/life*. For information about the Rethinking School Lunch/LiFE network, please visit *www.rethinkingschoollunch-life.org*.

TEACHERS COLLEGE
COLUMBIA UNIVERSITY

Teachers College Columbia University, Center for Food & Environment, 525 West 120th Street Box 137, New York, NY 10027

The National Gardening Association (NGA) is a nonprofit organization established in 1972. Its mission is to promote home, school, and community gardening as a means to renew and sustain the essential connection between people, plants, and the environment. NGA's programs and initiatives are targeted to five areas: plant-based education, health and wellness, environmental stewardship, community development, and responsible home gardening. For more information on NGA and its programs, please visit *www.garden.org* and *www.kidsgardening.org* or call (800) 538-7476.

Department of Health and Human Services • National Institutes of Health
Supported by a Science Education Partnership Award (SEPA) from the National Center for Research Resources
This publication was made possible by a Science Education Partnership Award (SEPA), grant number R25 RR12374 from the National Center for Research Resources (NCRR), a component of the National Institutes of Health (NIH). Its contents are solely the responsibility of the authors and do not necessarily represent the official views of NCRR or NIH.

Printed in the United States of America.

ISBN 978-0-915873-47-0

Library of Congress Control Number: 2007928840

Linking Food and the Environment Project Team

PRINCIPAL INVESTIGATOR
Isobel R. Contento, PhD, Mary Swartz Rose Professor of Nutrition Education, Teachers College Columbia University

CO-PRINCIPAL INVESTIGATOR
Angela Calabrese Barton, PhD, Associate Professor of Science Education, Michigan State University

AUTHOR AND PROJECT DIRECTOR
Pamela A. Koch, EdD, RD, Executive Director, Center for Food & Environment, Teachers College Columbia University

Growing Food Team

Author
Pamela A. Koch, EdD, RD

Lesson Development, Implementation, and Evaluation
Tracy Cullen, MS, RD
Marcia Dadds, MS, RD
Sumi Hagiwara, PhD
Stacia Helfand, MS, EdM, RD
Toby Jane Hindin, EdD
Ana De Lourdes Islas, EdD, RD
Meredith Smart, PhD
Michelle Trudeau, MA
Karen Wadsworth, EdD

Teacher Contributors
Steven Broder, MBA, MS, P.S. 50
Nicholas Graham, EdM, I.S. 528
Kathy Ortiz, Bilingual Bicultural Mini School

Advisors
Ronald DeMeersman, PhD, Human Physiology
Joan D. Gussow, EdD, Food Systems
Toni Liquori, EdD, Food Systems and Implementation Issues
Patricia Zybert, PhD, Statistician

Field Test Partners
Center for Ecoliteracy, Berkeley, CA, Zenobia Barlow, Executive Director
Environmental Education Council of Marin, San Rafael, CA, Sandy Wallenstein, Executive Director
The Food Trust, Philadelphia, PA, Sandra Sherman, EdD
Lawrence Hall of Science, Berkeley, CA, Katherine Barrett, PhD
University of Missouri, St. Louis, MO, William Kyle, PhD
University of Texas, Austin, TX, Julie Loft, PhD

Production Team

Editorial Director
Margo Crabtree

Editor
Loaiza Ortiz

Copy Editor
Kate Norris

Proofreader
Rachel Bartlett

Editorial Assistants
Karin Fliesch
Lauren Gellar

Original Design and Art Direction
Lisa Cicchetti

Design, Art Direction, and Page Layout
Alison Watt, National Gardening
  Association

Natural Science Illustration
Cornelia Blik

Icons and Editorial Illustration
Anne Faust

Photography
Zenobia Barlow, Center for Ecoliteracy
James Tyler, Center for Ecoliteracy

Page 113 Photo
Suzanne De John, National Gardening
  Association

Cover Photo
Zenobia Barlow and James Tyler,
  Center for Ecoliteracy
  *Students enjoy a spring harvest at
  The Edible Schoolyard, Martin Luther
  King, Jr. Middle School*

To all of the children who participate in *LiFE*
and to the future of our food supply.

Contents

UNIT 1: BECOMING FOOD SCIENTISTS

UNIT 2: PLANTS

UNIT 3: FOOD WEBS

UNIT 4: AGRICULTURE

UNIT 5: MAKING CHOICES

Illustrations

Acknowledgments

The seed for the LiFE Program was planted in the 1970s when Joan D. Gussow, EdD, the Mary Swartz Rose Professor of Nutrition Education Emeritus, brought the perspective of food-system study to Teachers College Columbia University. LiFE began with the simple goal of developing an inquiry-based science curriculum that would educate children about the relationship between food systems, food choice, and personal health. Because of the ideas, thoughts, and dedication of so many, the LiFE Curriculum Series has grown and expanded to include the interplay of biology, personal behavior, and the present food system and technological environment, which encourage over-consumption and sedentary behavior. It is our hope that the LiFE Curriculum Series will enhance students' personal motivation and competence to use their science understandings to reflect upon and purposefully act upon their world with the aim of transforming themselves and conditions of their lives.

Many people have been involved in the development of the *Growing Food* module of the LiFE Curriculum Series and we are indebted to them all. To those who have reviewed our materials, offered suggestions and insights, and shared experiences and challenges, we thank you. To the many educators and students who tested lessons and offered feed-back, we appreciate your enthusiasm for *Growing Food* and your valuable contributions. To our field-test school principals, teachers, and students, we thank you for working with us to make *Growing Food* what it is today. We learned so much from you. To our families and friends who have lived with this project for many years, we are deeply grateful for your warm support and endless patience.

2001–2004 Field-Test Partners

New York City Board of Education, New York, NY: Community School District 6

Center for Ecoliteracy, Berkeley, CA: Berkeley Unified School District

Food Trust, Philadelphia, PA: Philadelphia School District

Lawrence Hall of Science, Berkeley, CA: Hayward Unified School District and Mt. Diablo School District

University of Missouri, St. Louis, MO: Maplewood-Richmond Heights School District and Normandy School District

University of Texas, Austin, TX: Austin Independent School District

Natural Science Illustration

We are grateful to the following gardeners and farmers for literally pulling up whole plants to provide our illustrator, Cornelia Blik, with botanical specimens as reference material.

Clinton Blount and Margo Crabtree, Aptos, CA; Oscar and Peggy Crabtree, Ledgecroft, Bridgewater, CT; Henry Ference, Painter Ridge Farm, Roxbury, CT; and Jean-Paul Courtens and Jody Bolluyt, Roxbury Farm, Kinderhook, NY.

Introduction

Welcome! You and your students are about to embark on an exciting adventure — learning science through the study of our food-production system, from nature's intricate and amazing system to the human-designed agricultural system.

Human impact on the natural world is expected to increase as human populations grow and as science and technology develop ever more sophisticated ways to manage the natural world to meet human desires more effectively. Today's children, as tomorrow's adults, need solid understanding of science concepts and skills to engage in scientific discussions and to participate in public debate about important issues that involve science and technology. During their lifetimes, today's children will be called upon to make many decisions about their personal health, including how to choose foods that will lead to nutritional well-being.

Children are naturally curious. They are investigators and problem-solvers, attempting to understand the natural and designed worlds. They already are "doing science." They may not always be aware of that fact, since "science" is often thought of as content that is abstract from everyday life. But science can be made personally meaningful … and it is in *LiFE!* We hope this module of the LiFE Curriculum Series brings enjoyment, learning, and growth to you and your students.

Isobel Contento
Angela Calabrese Barton
Pamela Koch

Goals

Students who participate in *LiFE* will:

- **increase their knowledge and conceptual understandings** about how the biological world works and how it interacts with the human-designed world;

- **develop skills in scientific inquiry** about the natural and designed world; use evidence to justify statements; use both logical reasoning and imagination; and be able to explain, to predict, and to identify and limit bias;

- **expand their ways of thinking or habits of mind** to include curiosity, flexibility, open-mindedness, informed skepticism, creativity, and critical thinking;

- **improve their attitudes toward the processes of science** through enjoyable activities in a domain that is meaningful and familiar to them — food;

- **improve their attitudes toward the natural environment** that include an appreciation of nature's complexity, diversity, change, and constancy; respect for the natural environment; and concern for the impact of human food systems on the environment;

- **improve their attitudes toward their personal health** through an understanding of the impact of food on health and an appreciation of healthful eating habits;

- **appreciate the connectedness** of science, technology, the natural environment, and everyday life in ways that are life-changing for the students themselves, for society, and for the natural environment;

- **increase confidence and commitment** to apply the above conceptual understandings, skills, attitudes, and ways of thinking (habits of mind) to personal decisions and public debate of issues related to food systems, health, and the natural environment.

Making Science Real, Meaningful, and Successful

Children construct meanings about their environment through their explorations of the world around them all the time. Using their senses, they make observations and use those to make predictions about how things work. They use their developing understandings to build a complex framework for how the world works.

Yet children's explanations of the natural world are incomplete and sometimes even scientifically unsound. For example, from a scientific perspective, we know that living things are distinguished from nonliving things in their ability to carry on the following life processes: movement, metabolism, growth, responsiveness to environmental stimuli, and reproduction. However, many children believe that objects are living if they move or grow. For example, the sun, wind, and clouds are living because they move. Fires are living because they consume wood, move, require air, reproduce (sparks cause other fires), and give off waste (smoke). [1, 2]

As teachers, we need to continually remind ourselves that children build their personal scientific ideas over many years of explorations. Therefore, it is difficult, at best, for science teachers to help children "change" their understandings with one or two lessons. Children need time, as a whole class, in small groups, and individually, to think through new forms of evidence, new explanations, and new ideas alongside their preexisting ideas. For new ideas to take hold, they must not only make sense to students, but they should also "fit" the complex framework that children have created outside of the classroom.

Since the early 1970s, research on learning has shown us how important it is that we begin science instruction from the standpoint of students' experiences. David Ausubel[3] emphasized this by distinguishing between "meaningful learning" and "rote learning." For meaningful learning to occur, the learner must be able to relate new knowledge to relevant existing concepts in his or her cognitive structure. As the National Science Education Standards remind us, "In the same way that scientists develop their knowledge and understanding as they seek answers to questions about the natural world, students develop an understanding of the natural world when they are actively engaged in scientific inquiry — alone and with others." [4]

Despite these advances in our understanding of how children learn and its importance for how we teach, elementary and middle school science has not followed suit. Science is often taught as if students do not already have their own ideas about how the world works or as if their out-of-school experiences could be easily displaced by school knowledge. Yet we know from our own experiences and from the literature on misconceptions that children come to school with certain beliefs about how things happen and that these beliefs are tenacious. Unless, as teachers, we draw upon these experiences and connect what we are teaching to the students' worlds, we will make little headway with meaningful learning, and children's incomplete ideas will persist. Indeed, science-education research shows that many students complete elementary, middle, and even high school with strongly held misconceptions about core science concepts, like the flow of matter and energy in ecosystems (such as the food-making process or the release of energy from food), even though these core ideas are commonly taught and are covered in most middle school curricular materials. [5]

Why is this? There are many factors that shape how and why students are not learning science for deep conceptual understanding, including instruction, the curriculum, and the knowledge base of the teacher. However, most recently, the American Association for the Advancement of Science has shown how important curricular materials are. They show us that "while better curriculum materials alone are unlikely to improve student learning, high-quality curriculum materials can positively influence student learning directly and through their influence on teachers." [6] After all, nearly 90 percent of science teachers use curricular materials 95 percent of the time. [7]

AAAS has put forth a research-based framework for evaluating how well curricular materials support teachers and students in meaningful teaching and learning. Their framework is partly structured around the following:

- How well does the **content** of the curriculum align with the big ideas of science?

- How well does the **presentation of ideas** within the curriculum support a teacher's instructional approach in ways that help teachers take account of students' prior ideas?

- Are the suggestions for **assessment** aimed at specific benchmarks and standards that are likely to reveal what students actually know (as opposed to rote memorization of these goals)?

In the design of the LiFE Program, these three criteria are central. The topics covered in this module are about plants as the foundation of life, the flow of energy and matter, and how nature's biological system and our human-designed agricultural system work together to supply us with food. Information is presented for teachers to use in questioning students about their current understanding of the topics of study. This allows students to combine their current thinking with what they are learning to develop new knowledge constructs. Our assessments include activity sheets that challenge the students to collect thorough, accurate data and to carefully interpret these data, along with writing assignments in their LiFE Logs, to reflect on what they learned while expanding their thinking.

Common Misconceptions

There are several important misconceptions to be aware of connected to "How Nature Provides Us with Food."

Students may believe that:

- *Plants get food from soil and fertilizer.* Students may believe that plants get food to help them grow from soil and fertilizer. It is important to pay attention to how we talk about plants and what they need to grow. Calling fertilizer "plant food" may promote these misconceptions. Remind students that plants synthesize their own food through photosynthesis and that soil and fertilizer provide other elements important for healthy plants. [8]

- *Plants get energy from other sources besides the sun.* Connected to the misconception discussed above, students often believe that plants get energy to make food from soil, water, fertilizer, and minerals. However, plants only get energy from the sun. [9]

- *Anything going into a plant or organism is food, including sunlight, minerals, water, and carbon dioxide.* As discussed above, plants make their food, they do not take it up from soil, water, or sunlight, and the only source of energy for food production is the sun. [10]

- *Food chains are linear and unidirectional.* In textbook diagrams, food chains may often be represented in a linear way, which can lead to misconceptions. In reality, food chains are quite complex, multidirectional and nonlinear. [11]

- *Respiration is the same as breathing.* Students often understand biological processes in reference to animal/human processes, thus equating plant respiration with breathing in animals. In respiration, plants use oxygen to convert the sugar produced during photosynthesis back into energy for growth.

Avoid using words like "breathing," which refers only to how animals take up air into their lungs. [12]

- *Celery is a stem.* Celery is actually a stalk. The word "stalk" is short for "leafstalk," which makes sense since celery leaves are found at the end of each stalk. An easy way to distinguish stems from stalks is to remember that stems are either circular or square in cross section. If you remove all the celery stalks you will find a short, conically shaped stem at the base. [13]

- *Seasonal diets are not nutritionally adequate.* People unfamiliar with seasonal diets may believe that it is difficult to get an adequate supply of essential nutrients from foods available locally year-round. In reality, largely seasonal diets, complemented by foods that have been preserved, provide more than an adequate supply of calories and nutrients. [14]

- *All or almost all foods grow in all climactic regions.* Again, if students are unfamiliar with regional food supplies they may not realize that different foods grow in different climates. This misconception is exacerbated by the abundance represented in supermarkets, where students may be led to believe that bananas grow in North Dakota! [15]

[1] Driver, Squires, Rushworth, & Wood-Robinson, 1994
[2] Kyle & Shymansky, 1989
[3] Ausubel, 1968
[4] NSES, 1996, p. 27
[5] Stern & Roseman, 2004
[6] Stern & Roseman, 2004, p. 539
[7] Renner, Abraham, Grzybowski, & Marek, 1990
[8] Goh, Yoke-Kum, & Lian-Sai, 1993
[9] Anderson, Sheldon, & DuBay, 1990
[10] Driver et al., 1994
[11] Anderson et al., 1990
[12] Driver et al., 1994
[13] Hershey, 2004
[14] Wilkins, Bowdish, & Sobal, 2002
[15] Wilkins, Bowdish, & Sobal, 2002

Getting Acquainted with *Growing Food*

Throughout this module, you and your students will investigate the question, *How does nature provide us with food?* This question is more complicated than it may seem. In this module, you and your students will learn more about human reliance on ecosystems and you'll begin to explore the impact of human activity on the natural world.

As you begin your investigations, you'll find yourself immersed in a world of complex systems. There is the Earth system, there are ecosystems, and there are food systems, to name just a few. Earth is home to many biotic (living) and abiotic (nonliving) things. Humans play a unique role in ecosystems in that we rely on both the natural world and the designed (human-managed) world for survival, including meeting our food needs. Where once we lived according to the seasons, with the aid of technology we now can grow crops in deserts, ship fresh foods around the world, and have access to fresh fruits and vegetables year-round. These accomplishments are possible only with sophisticated farming techniques, highly technological food processing factories, and extensive transportation systems.

As part of a complex biological system, humans have responsibilities to the other parts of our system. To insure our own survival, we must respect the wide diversity of living creatures — both large and small — and the physical components that all life depends on for growth and sustainability. Our planet has limited resources that cannot be carelessly wasted or polluted without running the risk of jeopardizing life on Earth. By investigating this module's question, your students will become informed citizens, prepared to make choices that will help support a sustainable future for generations to come.

If you have access to a school garden, we encourage you to engage your students in growing their own food. Gardens also can serve as living laboratories where students can set up investigations and monitor them over time. Gardens are a great place to monitor the effects of changing weather conditions on garden ecosystems, decomposition, the seed-to-table life cycle

of garden plants, and much more. The National Gardening Association's Web site (*www.kidsgardening.org*) is an excellent resource for both ideas and materials.

Overview
This module consists of five units, each with its own driving question.

Unit 1
Becoming Food Scientists introduces LiFE and explores the question, *What is a food scientist?* Investigating corn motivates students to study food. Studying grapes introduces students to LiFE's QuESTA Learning Cycle. Assessing what students already know about how nature provides us with food offers a baseline to track student growth throughout this module.

Unit 2
Plants introduces students to complex biological systems through the question, *If there were no plants, would humans have food?* Students set up plant experiments to explore energy transformations and learn about the process of photosynthesis. A lesson about food chains helps students understand how much living things depend on plants.

Unit 3
Food Webs builds on what students have learned about producer-consumer interactions and introduces decomposers through the question, *How do components in nature interact with each other?* Students explore the process of decomposition in nature, build a classroom compost bin, and complete the unit by creating their own food web diagrams.

Unit 4
Agriculture takes students from the natural world to the human-designed system for producing the plants and animals we eat. The Unit Question, *How do we interact with nature to meet our food needs?* leads students through investigations of the ways humans depend on farmers for our food. Students plant classroom crops to try their hand at being farmers.

Unit 5

Making Choices guides students through the process of making informed decisions by asking, *How can we use the science we learned to make food and agriculture choices?* Students explore regional food systems, compare different farming practices, design a farm, and reflect on all they have learned by revisiting the Module Question, *How does nature provide us with food?*

Promoting Inquiry

Teaching science as inquiry makes science a process of doing and thinking instead of learning a set of predetermined facts. This changes your role as teacher. Instead of being a source of science facts, you are a partner with your students as you seek answers or explanations. It means turning students' questions back on them. If a student asks, *What happens to plants that don't get light?* respond with, *Well, I'm not sure. How shall we find out?* This sends a powerful message — that knowing how to find an answer is as important as knowing the answer.

Ask open-ended questions that promote reflection and further questions. "How" and "why" questions work well: *Why do you think that is?* or *How would we find out?* Ask questions that encourage critical thinking, like: *What evidence or observation leads you to that conclusion?* Help your students develop theories and bring closure to their explorations and experiments by asking: *How would you explain your results?* and *What theories can you think of to explain this?*

QuESTA Learning Cycle

How students learn is as important as what they learn in the LiFE curriculum. The questions that drive the modules and units in LiFE challenge students to explore, question, investigate, analyze, synthesize, and act. LiFE's five-phase learning cycle, QuESTA, guides students through this process.

EXPERIMENTING

Students plan and conduct experiments to answer the questions within the area of study. Thus, students identify problems, state hypotheses, select methods, display results, and draw conclusions from these experiments to further their knowledge.

SEARCHING

Students seek out other information already known about their topic through readings provided in the lessons, researching in the library, or on the computer, and interviewing people.

THEORIZING

Through thoughtful reflection and synthesis of what they have learned in the previous phases, the students develop their own theories and constructs about how the world works. Students gain skills that enable them to articulate theories, give evidence to support their arguments, and appropriately challenge the theories of others.

APPLYING TO LIFE

Students apply the new constructs and processes they learned through the unit to decisions and actions they make each day. Students develop new questions to continue their exploration in the area of study. This phase of QuESTA also is an opportunity for you and your students to extend the LiFE activities. For example, in Lesson 2 as students learn about grapes, you may wish to have students investigate what climate grapes grow in, where the grapes they buy in their local market are grown, and how far they have to travel to reach the market. Look for ideas for going further on the LiFE Web site.

Using QuESTA

The activities that focus on questioning, experimenting, and searching are engaging and often easy to implement in the classroom. Activities that call for students to theorize and apply to life help students refine their abilities to construct explanations and theories about what they have learned from their exploring and experimenting and to apply their learning to their

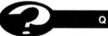

QUESTIONING

Students explore their prior knowledge and experiences related to the area of study and develop and refine meaningful questions to guide further inquiry. They also share their current conceptions about the topic so that any misconceptions can be addressed.

QUESTA PHASES AND ASSOCIATED TERMS

This table includes terms for each phase of QuESTA. We developed this to help you and your students understand and differentiate among the types of action or activities appropriate for each phase. These terms are used throughout the teacher and student materials.

QUESTIONING	EXPERIMENTING	SEARCHING	THEORIZING	APPLYING TO LIFE
assess	check	discover	analyze	apply
assess knowledge	conduct	explore	build theories	carry out
consider	create research	find out	compare	embark
contemplate	questions	gain knowledge	conclude	employ
inquire	designing	about	construct	implement
mull over	experiments	learn about	knowledge	put into action
ponder	determine	look into	contrast	undertake
pose	displaying data	research	create ideas	use
question	evaluate	search	debate	utilize
speculate	examine	seek	deliberate	
think about	experiment		discuss	
wonder	gather data		envision	
	hypothesize		explain	
	inspect		imagine	
	identify variable		infer	
	investigate		realize	
	manipulate		reason	
	observe		recognize	
	predict		reflect	
	probe		summarize	
	prove		think through	
	solve			
	study			
	test			

daily lives. Pay special attention to the theorizing and application activities in the lessons. These activities will help you meet some important and challenging standards. The National Science Education Standards and the AAAS Project 2061 Benchmarks suggest that in addition to making observations and designing and conducting investigations, students should:

- use logical reasoning and critical thinking to link evidence with explanations;

- use communication skills to describe observations, summarize results, articulate theories and constructs about how the world works, consider alternative explanations, and challenge the explanations proposed by others;

- apply scientific constructs and processes to everyday decisions and actions.

Assessment Strategies

Authentic assessment tasks provide students with opportunities to construct meaning from what they have learned. The LiFE Curriculum Series offers different assessment strategies to help you track your students' progress. Many of these are integrated into the lessons.

Pre-Assessment

Lesson 4 serves as this module's pre-assessment. Students answer the Module Question, *How does nature provide us with food?* As students respond to this question, remind them that they will not be graded on their answers. Encourage students to write down what they know and think now.

Post-Assessment

In Lesson 20, students revisit the Module Question, look at their responses to the question in the pre-assessment, and reflect on what they have learned. Make this post-assessment an exciting academic challenge for your students. As a teacher you not only want your students to know the content taught; you want them to be able to use their knowledge and skills in the real world.

Ongoing Assessment

Throughout the module, students have multiple opportunities to participate in full class discussions, and to work and discuss materials in small groups and present their work to the class. These interactions offer opportunities to assess how students are thinking about the topics being studied, their level of sophistication in what they are thinking and saying, and their abilities to engage in discussions, debates, and scientific arguments with their peers. These ongoing assessments may be particularly helpful for students who are challenged by writing and public speaking. In each lesson, students write in their LiFE Logs, reflecting on what they have learned. This reflective writing gives students the freedom to express in their own words what they are learning in class. Often the LiFE Log assignment will be an answer to an open-ended question, which will help you assess how students have internalized what they learned in the lessons, how they made meaning of new concepts, and how they brought former ideas to bear on new understandings.

How to Use This Book

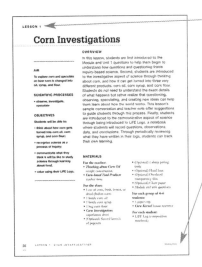

Header: This indicates the type of page. For example, a Lesson Plan, Teacher Note, Lesson Resource, Sample Conversation, Student Reading, Experiment Sheet, or Activity Sheet.

Footer: The lesson number, title, and page number are shown at the bottom of each page.

Units: The module's unit titles are listed in order down the side of the page. The name of the unit you are working with is shown in bold type.

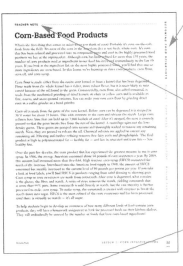

Teacher Pages: Teacher pages, such as the Teacher Note, are distinguished by the absence of a QuESTA icon.

Student Pages: All student pages include a QuESTA icon indicating the phase of the QuESTA learning cycle that corresponds with the activity students are engaged in. For example, the Searching icon appears on the Reading for LiFE pages. All student pages are designed to be copied for use as handouts.

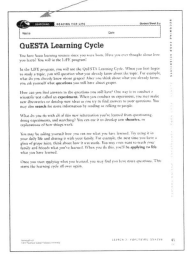

Each lesson includes teacher materials and most lessons have student materials. The teacher materials include a lesson plan and additional information written for the teacher. We recommend reviewing these materials as you do prep for the lesson. The student materials include readings and activity sheets.

LESSON FORMAT

Each lesson contains an activity and supplemental materials that support the activity. These materials will include any background information, teaching suggestions, illustrations, student readings, and student activity sheets that are needed to teach the lesson. While the lessons appear in a specific order in the module, we encourage you to think about your students' needs and abilities and to adjust the order of the lessons accordingly. For example, we found students were motivated to learn more about plant parts after they made the plant parts salad. However, you may wish to teach your class about plants parts before making the salad. Either way works. The descriptions below highlight the type of information you will find in the lessons.

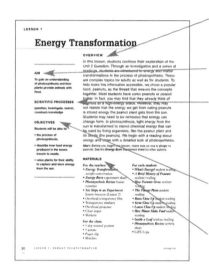

Overview: This section provides a description of the lesson and details both what the students will do and what they will learn from the lesson.

Aim: This summarizes the main idea of the lesson.

Scientific Processes: These terms are related to specific phases of the QuESTA learning cycle. They indicate which QuESTA phases are emphasized in the lesson and the skills that students will be using as they complete the activity.

Objectives: These highlight what you can expect your students to know and be able to do at the end of the lesson.

Materials: This lists the recommended materials for the lesson. For your convenience, there is a materials list for the entire module on pages 21–22 that includes general materials used in many of the lessons, as well as lesson-specific materials. Materials listed in **_bold italics_** are teacher and student pages provided in this book.

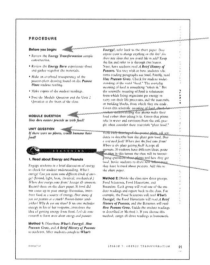

Before You Begin: Some activities require advance preparation. You may need to make copies of reproducibles, gather materials, post the Module and Unit questions, or review the teacher note or sample conversation.

Module Question: Each lesson lists the Module Question.

Unit Question: Each lesson lists the Unit Question.

Lesson Procedure: The lesson procedure provides step-by-step information to complete the lesson. QuESTA icons used throughout the procedure indicate which phase of the QuESTA Learning Cycle is being emphasized. Each lesson begins by engaging students in the concept. Each lesson opens with an opportunity for you to check for student understanding, review the Module Question, and introduce or review the Unit Question.

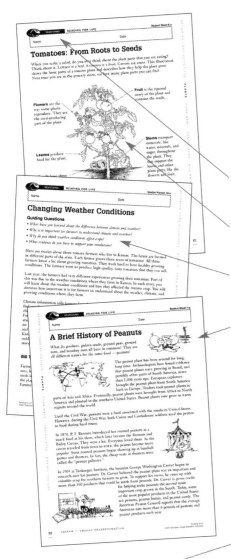

STUDENT PAGES

These reproducibles include student readings and activity sheets.

Reading for Life

An **icon** represents the phase in the QuESTA Learning Cycle that the reading addresses.

Detailed **natural science illustrations** help students gain a deeper understanding of the topic.

Guiding questions help students organize the new information they are learning.

Editorial art makes the page more engaging to a student audience and helps communicate the reading's ideas.

Activity Sheets

These pages help students focus their learning and guide student data collection and analysis. They provide questions to guide student thinking and help students reflect on what they have learned. Completed activity sheets can help you assess student learning as you progress through each unit.

SUPPLEMENTAL TEACHER MATERIAL

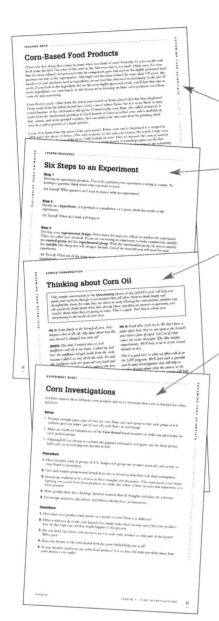

Teacher Notes include helpful background information.

Lesson Resources provide information that supports conducting the activity.

Sample Conversations demonstrate the level of thinking and discussion recommended for students to reflect on what they learned in order to develop new theories from the activity.

Experiment Sheets provide a detailed description of the set-up, procedure, and questions to guide class discussion.

Materials

The materials listed below include general materials that will be used throughout the module, specific materials required for each lesson, and teacher resources and student materials provided in this manual.

General materials

Chart paper
Markers
Crayons
Overhead projector
Overhead transparency film
Transparency marker
Hand lenses
Scissors
Napkins or paper towels
LiFE Logs (one composition notebook for each student)

Lesson-specific materials

UNIT 1: BECOMING FOOD SCIENTISTS

Lesson 1: Corn Investigations
1 ear of corn, fresh, frozen, or dried (Indian corn)
1 bottle corn oil
1 bottle corn syrup
1 bag corn flour
(Optional) Several kernels of popcorn
(Optional) 1 sharp paring knife
1 paper cup for each group of 4–6 students

Lesson 2: Exploring Grapes
3–4 grapes per student

Lesson 3: Making Grape Juice
3 bunches of grapes
Materials as listed for class experiment from Lesson 2

Lesson 4: Pre-Assessment
2 houseplants (geraniums work well)
Aluminum foil
4 paper clips
2 pebbles
2 clear plastic bags
Petroleum jelly
Tape or twist ties
1 large white index card per student

UNIT 2: PLANTS

Lesson 6: Celebrating Plant Parts
2 basic white paper plates per student
1 plastic knife and fork per student
1 sharp knife for chopping
1 vegetable peeler
1 cutting board
3 serving spoons
1 whisk

3–6 small bowls
3 large bowls
1 colander
1 head lettuce, romaine or other dark-green lettuce
1 bag mixed salad greens
7 carrots
1 bunch celery
1 bunch broccoli
1 pint cherry tomatoes, or 7 larger tomatoes
8 ounces ready-to-eat sunflower seeds
Olive oil
Red vinegar
Honey
Dijon mustard
2 shallots
2 cloves garlic
Salt and pepper

Lesson 7: Energy Transformation
5 dry-roasted peanuts
1 potato
Paper clip
Matches

Lesson 8: Linking Plants and Animals
5 skeins of different colored yarn
Pushpins
5 index cards
5 red or orange markers
5 blue or black markers

UNIT 3: FOOD WEBS

Lesson 9: Nature's Decomposers
Compost bin — you can buy a pre-made bin or make your own. To make your own, see the *Making a Compost Bin* lesson resource.

Lesson 10: Classroom Composting
Compost bin from Lesson 9
Shredded newspaper
Spray bottle with water
1 pound red wiggler worms
1–2 pounds food scraps

UNIT 4: AGRICULTURE

Lesson 12: No Farmers, No Food
1 apple

Lesson 13: Classroom Crops
5 planters, 24"–36" long
Soil
Compost

Seeds
Watering can
Masking tape
(Optional) wooden plant markers

Lesson 14: Investigating Soil
8–10 cups soil from a place where plants are growing
8–10 cups soil from a place where no plants are growing
20 paper plates

Lesson 15: Soil Texture
2 clear 1-quart glass or plastic jars with secure lids
Water
Spray bottle with water
Two labels
2 cups or handfuls of soil
10 paper towels or paper plates

UNIT 5: MAKING CHOICES

Lesson 17: Regional Eating
Fruits and/or vegetables (or pictures of them) corresponding to each region for whatever season it is currently
Wall map of the United States
Thumbtacks
(Optional) fruits and/or vegetables from a farmer's market or other local source. Try bringing foods you think the students might not be familiar with, if possible.

Lesson 18: Comparing Farming Practices
(Optional) sample newspapers, newsletters, or time lines for reference

Lesson 19: Frieda Farmer's Design Project
(Optional) magazines with photographs of farms or large vegetable gardens

Lesson 20: Bringing It All Together
1 large index card per student

Teacher resources and student materials provided in this manual

UNIT 1: BECOMING FOOD SCIENTISTS

Lesson 1: Corn Investigations
Thinking about Corn Oil sample conversation

Science Standards Matrices

National Science Education Standards
to be met by the end of 8th grade*

	GROWING FOOD UNITS				
	UNIT 1 **Becoming Food Scientists**	UNIT 2 Plants	UNIT 3 Food Webs	UNIT 4 Agriculture	UNIT 5 **Making Choices**
A. SCIENCE AS INQUIRY					
1. Abilities necessary to do scientific inquiry	X	X	X	X	X
2. Understandings about scientific inquiry	X	X	X	X	
C. LIFE SCIENCE					
1. Structure and Function in Living Systems					
2. Reproduction and Heredity					
3. Regulation and Behavior					
4. Populations and Ecosystems		X	X	X	
5. Diversity and Adaptations of Organisms					
E SCIENCE AND TECHNOLOGY					
1. Abilities of Technological Design					
2. Understandings about Science and Technology				X	X
F. SCIENCE IN PERSONAL AND SOCIAL PERSPECTIVES					
1. Personal Health					X
2. Populations, Resources, and Environments				X	X
3. Natural Hazards				X	X
4. Risks and Benefits					X
5. Science and Technology in Society				X	X
6. Science as a Human Endeavor	X	X	X	X	X
G. HISTORY AND NATURE OF SCIENCE					
1. Nature of Science	X	X	X	X	X

*National Research Council (1996). See full text of the standards at *www.nap.edu/readingroom/books/nses/html/6d.html*

KEY: **XX** Fully covers **X** Touches upon

Benchmarks for Science Literacy
to be met by the end of 8th grade*

GROWING FOOD UNITS

	UNIT 1 Becoming Food Scientists	UNIT 2 Plants	UNIT 3 Food Webs	UNIT 4 Agriculture	UNIT 5 Making Choices
1. THE NATURE OF SCIENCE					
A. The Scientific World	X	X	X	X	X
B. Scientific Inquiry	XX	XX	X	X	X
C. The Scientific Enterprise	X	X	X		
3. THE NATURE OF TECHNOLOGY					
A. Technology and Science					X
B. Design and Systems				X	X
C. Issues in Technology				X	X
5. THE LIVING ENVIRONMENT					
A. Diversity of Life		X	X		
B. Heredity					
C. Cells					
D. Interdependence of Life		X	X	X	
E. Flow of Matter and Energy		X	X	X	
F. Evolution of Life					
7. HUMAN SOCIETY					
A. Cultural Effects on Behavior				X	X
B. Group Behavior					
C. Social Change				X	X
D. Social Trade-offs				X	X
E. Political and Economic Systems				X	X
F. Social Conflict					
G. Global Interdependence				X	X
8. THE DESIGNED WORLD					
A. Agriculture	X			XX	XX
B. Materials and Manufacturing	X			X	
C. Energy Sources and Use		X		X	X
D. Communication					
E. Information Processing					
F. Health Technology					
11. COMMON THEMES					
A. Systems		X	X	X	X
B. Models			X		
C. Constancy and Change			X	X	
D. Scale				X	X
12. HABITS OF MIND					
A. Values and Attitudes	X	XX	X	X	X
B. Computation and Estimation					
C. Manipulation and Observation					
D. Communication Skills			X		XX
E. Critical-Response Skills	X	X	X	X	X

*American Association for the Advancement of Science (1993). See full text of the standards at
www.project2061.org/publications/bsl/online/bolintro.htm

KEY: **XX** Fully covers **X** Touches upon

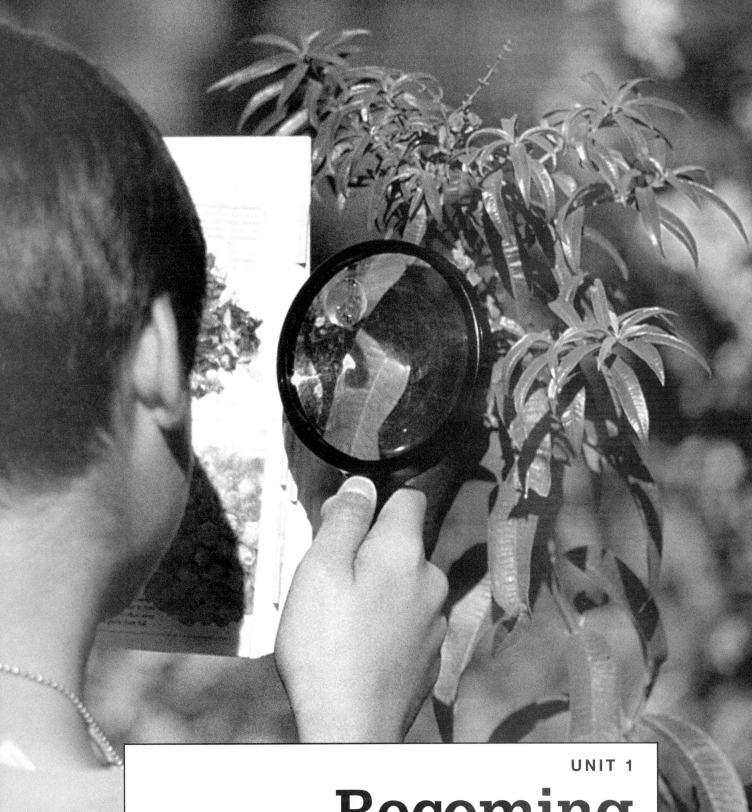

Becoming Food Scientists

Corn Investigations

AIM

To explore corn and speculate on how corn is changed into oil, syrup, and flour.

SCIENTIFIC PROCESSES

- observe, investigate, speculate

OBJECTIVES

Students will be able to:

- think about how corn gets turned into corn oil, corn syrup, and corn flour;

- recognize science as a process of inquiry;

- communicate what they think it will be like to study science through learning about food;

- value using their LiFE Logs.

OVERVIEW

In this lesson, students are first introduced to the Module and Unit 1 questions to help them begin to understand how questions and questioning frame inquiry-based science. Second, students are introduced to the investigative aspect of science through thinking about corn, and how it can get turned into three very different products: corn oil, corn syrup, and corn flour. Students do not need to understand the exact details of what happens but rather realize that questioning, observing, speculating, and creating new ideas can help them learn about how the world works. This lesson's sample conversation and teacher note offer suggestions to guide students through this process. Finally, students are introduced to the communicative aspect of science through being introduced to LiFE Logs, a notebook where students will record questions, observations, data, and conclusions. Through periodically reviewing what they have written in their logs, students can track their own learning.

MATERIALS

For the teacher:
- *Thinking about Corn Oil* sample conversation
- *Corn-Based Food Products* teacher note

For the class:
- 1 ear of corn, fresh, frozen, or dried (Indian corn)
- 1 bottle corn oil
- 1 bottle corn syrup
- 1 bag corn flour
- *Corn Investigations* experiment sheet
- (Optional) Several kernels of popcorn

- (Optional) 1 sharp paring knife
- (Optional) Hand lens
- (Optional) Overhead transparency film
- (Optional) Chart paper
- Module and Unit questions

For each group of 4–6 students:
- 1 paper cup
- *Corn Kernel* lesson resource

For each student:
- LiFE Log (composition notebook)

PROCEDURE

Before You Begin:

- Follow the setup instructions on the *Corn Investigations* experiment sheet.

- Review the *Thinking about Corn Oil* sample conversation and the *Corn-Based Food Products* teacher note.

- Make copies of the *Corn Kernel* lesson resource to distribute to each group of students.

- Post the Module Question and the Unit 1 Question at the front of the classroom.

MODULE QUESTION

How does nature provide us with food?

UNIT QUESTION

What is a food scientist?

 QUESTIONING

1. Introduce LiFE

Explain to students that they are about to begin a science program that focuses on the study of food. In LiFE, your students are scientists — a special kind of scientist called a food scientist. *What do you think food scientists might do? What kind of knowledge do they need?* Accept all answers. Record students' ideas on chart paper or on the board.

Food scientists investigate food in lots of different ways. Some study how food is produced. Others might look at how a food, like corn, is changed and combined with other foods to make another kind of food, like cereal, or cake, or pizza. There are food scientists who try to understand how what we eat influences our personal health. And there are food scientists who investigate how the waste and pollution created through growing, processing, and packaging our food affects our natural environment.

2. Discuss Module and Unit Questions

Post the Module Question and the Unit 1 Question on the board. Invite volunteers to read the questions out loud. Tell students that as LiFE food scientists, they will be investigating answers to questions like these.

Understanding what food scientists do will help students be better prepared for their work as LiFE food scientists. Make sure you give your students time to discuss their ideas about a food scientist's work. As students work through this lesson, check to see how their understanding has changed.

3. Explain and Conduct Corn Investigation

Show students the ear of corn and the ingredients made from corn: corn oil, corn syrup, and corn flour. *How do corn kernels get changed into corn oil, corn syrup, and corn flour?*

Follow the procedure outline on the *Corn Investigations* experiment sheet. Challenge students to think about different ways that corn gets changed into other products. Create a sense of mystery and intrigue. Make it clear that all ideas and thoughts are welcome. Remind students that they are asking questions and wondering about the products. They are not trying to come up with a correct answer. The sample conversation and teacher note can help you guide your students through this inquiry. Be sure to review the questions on the experiment sheet.

4. Have Groups Share Findings

Encourage a whole class conversation led by students. You may wish to have each group select a reporter to share the group's thoughts with the class. Remind students that this activity is about thinking, exploring, and learning. It is not about finding the correct answer. As the discussion comes to a close, remind students that as food scientists they are going to be investigating, experimenting, and developing new ideas about lots of topics related to food.

(Optional) Distribute the cut-up popcorn kernels to each group of students. Have students look at the inside of the kernel. The small core part near the bottom is called the germ. There is oil in the germ. The germ is the part that is squeezed to get out the oil. Invite students to try to rub the germ on paper. *Do you see a stain? What does that tell you?*

5. Discuss Science Inquiry

Explain that the corn investigation is an example of a science inquiry. *What do you think "science inquiry" means?*

After several students have shared their ideas, review this definition of **science inquiry**: using your own curiosity about a topic to help you put together what you already know with what you are learning to construct new knowledge that you can use in your daily life.

6. Introduce the LiFE Logs

Throughout *Growing Food,* students will keep a log to record thoughts, observations, data, and conclusions about what they are learning. This allows students to reflect on what they learn and to understand how their thinking grows and changes.

7. LiFE Logs

Write a paragraph about "What I think it will be like to be a food scientist."

If your students are not accustomed to this type of reflective writing, they may find it challenging. Help students understand that it is fine to sit in front of a blank page for a few moments as they think about what they want to write.

You may wish to brainstorm a list of ideas (as a whole class or individually) to serve as prompts. Students can use this list as they write their paragraphs.

8. Assign Homework

Have students write two questions in their LiFE Logs that reflect what they would like to learn about food.

Have students look at home and select five different kinds of food. Have them look at the ingredient lists to see if they can identify any ingredients made from corn. They can make a simple table, like the one shown below, in their LiFE Logs. Make sure students know how to read an ingredient list. You may wish to demonstrate in class.

Name of the Food	Ingredients from Corn in This Food

Thinking about Corn Oil

> This sample conversation in the **Questioning** phase of the QuESTA cycle will help you guide your students through a conversation that will allow them to think deeply and thoughtfully about the topic they are about to study. During the conversation, students may ask questions, think about what they already know, speculate on answers to questions, and wonder about what they are going to learn. This is a guide. Feel free to adjust your questioning to the needs of your class.

MS. D: Look closely at the kernels of corn. Now compare that to the oil. *Any ideas about how the corn kernel is changed into corn oil?*

JESSIE: One time I noticed that we had sunflower seed oil at my home. I asked my dad how the sunflower oil gets made from the seeds because I didn't see any oil in the seeds. He said the sunflower seeds are squeezed very hard and the oil comes out. Maybe if we squeeze the corn kernels very hard oil will come out.

MS. D: That's an interesting comparison to sunflower seeds. We can try squeezing one of our corn kernels. *What do you think would happen?*

ALEX: The corn kernel seems watery to me. I don't think water and oil are the same. I think if we squeeze a corn kernel, we will get wet, juicy stuff out, not oil. *How can we get oil from corn?*

MS. D: Good thinking. Let's start by figuring out how we can tell if we get water or oil from the corn. *Does anyone know how we can tell if what we get from squeezing a corn kernel is wet, juicy stuff or oil?*

ROSANNA: When I get pizza my mom always says that the stuff that gets on the paper plate and stains it is oil. If we squeeze the stuff that comes out of a corn kernel onto a paper plate and it's oil, it will stain the paper plate.

MS. D: Good idea. Let's try it. We don't have a paper plate here, but we can squeeze the kernel's juice onto a piece of paper. Let's see if what comes out stains the paper. (Do this simple experiment.) We'll have to let it sit for several minutes to dry.

This is a good start to what we often will do in the LiFE program. We'll start with a question and do some investigations that will help us develop theories about what the answer to the question might be. Our class discussions will help us come up with ideas. Talking through our ideas, even if your idea seems silly at first, is much more important than knowing the right answer. Scientists do this type of thinking and discussing all the time. Don't worry if you don't completely understand how corn flour, corn oil, and corn syrup are made from corn. You all did some excellent thinking about how corn gets changed. I think doing science this way is fun. I hope you do, too.

Continue the conversation to include a discussion of how corn kernels are made into corn syrup and corn flour.

Corn Investigations

Students observe three different corn products and try to determine how corn is changed into these products.

Setup

1. Prepare enough paper cups of corn oil, corn flour, and corn syrup so that each group of 4–6 students gets one paper cup of corn oil, corn flour, or corn syrup.

2. Make an overhead transparency of the *Corn Kernel* lesson resource or make one photocopy for each student group.

3. (Optional) If you choose to examine the popcorn endosperm and germ, use the sharp paring knife and cut several popcorn kernels in half.

Procedure

1. Have students work in groups of 4–6. Assign each group one product (corn oil, corn syrup, or corn flour) to investigate.

2. Give each student group several kernels from the ear of corn to help them with their investigation.

3. Encourage students to be creative in their thoughts and discussion. This experiment is not about figuring out exactly how these products are made, but rather to have an enjoyable experience as a food scientist.

4. Have groups share their findings. Remind students that all thoughts and ideas are welcome.

5. Encourage questions, discussion, and debates during these presentations.

Questions

1. How does your product look similar to a kernel of corn? How is it different?

2. What could you do to the corn kernels that might make them become more like your product? List all the steps you can that might happen in this process.

3. Do you think the whole corn kernel is used to make your product or only part of the kernel? What part?

4. Does the picture of the corn kernel with the parts labeled help you at all?

5. Is your product similar to any other food product? If it is, does this help you think about how your product was made?

Corn Kernel

The **seed coat** is mostly fiber and protects the kernel.

The space between the seed coat and the endosperm is the **air cavity.**

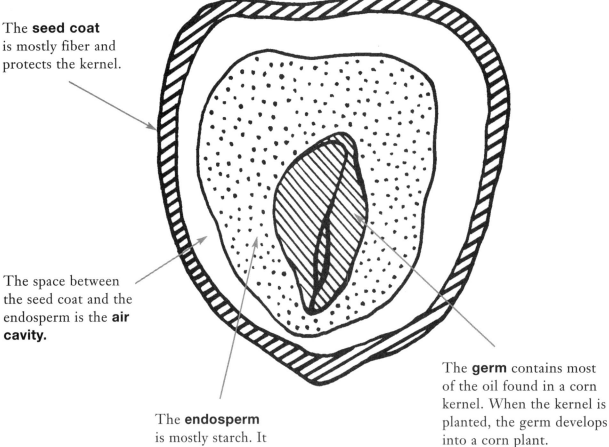

The **germ** contains most of the oil found in a corn kernel. When the kernel is planted, the germ develops into a corn plant.

The **endosperm** is mostly starch. It provides food for the young corn plant.

DID YOU KNOW . . . ?

A corn kernel is
16% water
 4% oil
20% fiber and protein
60% starch

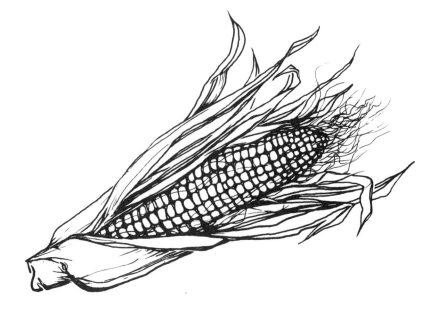

Corn-Based Food Products

What's the first thing that comes to mind when you think of corn? Probably it's corn-on-the-cob, fresh from the field. Yet most of the corn in the American diet is not fresh, whole corn. It's corn that has been refined and processed into its component parts and used in the highly processed food products we buy at the supermarket. Although corn has been refined for more than 150 years, the number of corn products used as ingredients in our food has increased tremendously in the last 50 years. If you look at the ingredient list on the most highly processed foods, you'll find that one or more ingredients are corn-based. In this lesson we're focusing on three corn products: corn flour, corn oil, and corn syrup.

Corn flour is made either from the entire corn kernel or from a kernel that has been degermed. Flour made from the whole kernel has a richer, more robust flavor, but it is more likely to turn rancid because of the oil found in the germ. Commercially, corn flour, also called cornmeal, is made from the mechanical grinding of dried kernels of white or yellow corn and is available in fine, coarse, and stone-ground varieties. You can make your own corn flour by grinding dried corn in a coffee grinder or a hand grinder.

Corn oil is made from the germ of the corn kernel. Before corn can be degermed it is steeped in 50°F water for about 35 hours. This adds moisture to the corn and releases the starch. Large corn refiners have bins that can hold up to 3,000 bushels of corn! After it's steeped, the corn is coarsely ground so that the germ breaks free from the rest of the kernel. A centrifuge spins out the low-density germs. These germs are pumped onto screens and thoroughly washed to remove any remaining starch. Next, they are pressed to release the oil. Chemical solvents are applied to extract any remaining oil. Filtering and further refining removes free fatty acids and phospholipids. The final product is high in polyunsaturated fat — healthy fat — and low in saturated and trans fats — less healthy fats.

Over the past few decades, the corn product that has experienced the greatest increase in use is corn syrup. In 1966 the average American consumed about 14 pounds of corn sweeteners a year. By 2004 this amount had increased more than five-fold. High fructose corn syrup (HFCS) accounted for much of the increase. Introduced into the American food supply in 1968, the amount of HFCS consumed has steadily increased to the current level of 80 pounds per person per year. If you take a look at food labels, you'll find HFCS in products ranging from salad dressing to chewing gum. Corn syrup or corn sweeteners are made from cornstarch. After corn is degermed, what remains is the gluten, the fiber, and starch. A series of steps removes the starch, yielding cornstarch that is more than 99% pure. Some cornstarch is sold directly as starch, but the vast majority is further processed to make corn syrup. To make syrup, the cornstarch is treated with enzymes to break the starch down into sugar. HFCS is the most refined of the corn sweeteners and has been processed until there is virtually no starch — it's all sugar.

To help students begin to develop an awareness of how many different kinds of food contain corn products, they will have a homework assignment to look for processed foods on their kitchen shelves. They will undoubtedly be amazed by the number of foods that have corn-based ingredients!

Exploring Grapes

AIM

To demonstrate the first three phases of QuESTA through observing and experimenting with grapes.

SCIENTIFIC PROCESSES

- **question, observe, investigate, hypothesize**

OBJECTIVES

Students will be able to:

- **describe new things they learned about grapes through carefully observing them;**

- **outline the steps of a procedure to turn grapes into grape juice;**

- **define the phases of the QuESTA Learning Cycle in their own words;**

- **express, in writing, what they have learned about grapes.**

OVERVIEW

Students are introduced to another key feature of LiFE — the QuESTA Learning Cycle. QuESTA has five phases: Questioning, Experimenting, Searching, Theorizing, and Applying to Life. This lesson covers the first three phases; Lesson 3 covers the remaining two. To gain an understanding of the way QuESTA guides the learning process, students participate in activities that take them through Questioning, Experimenting, and Searching. Students conduct detailed observations of grapes. Based on their observations, they pose questions to help them learn even more about grapes. They work in small groups to develop a procedure to change grapes into grape juice. Then they come together as scientists to discuss and debate their experiment procedures and reach consensus on a class procedure for making grape juice in the next lesson. Students experience the Searching phase as they read more about QuESTA. In their LiFE Logs, they summarize what they learned about grapes.

MATERIALS

For the teacher:
- *QuESTA!* lesson resource
- *Six Steps to an Experiment* lesson resource
- *Grapes and Grape Juice* teacher note
- *Scientific Inquiry* teacher note

For the class:
- Chart paper
- Markers

For each student:
- 3–4 grapes
- Napkins or paper towels
- *QuESTA Learning Cycle* student reading
- *Grape Explorations* activity sheet
- *Grape Experiment* activity sheet
- LiFE Log

PROCEDURE

Before You Begin:

- Review the background information in the *Grapes and Grape Juice* and *Scientific Inquiry* teacher notes.

- Detach and wash grapes, 3–4 per student

- Make copies of the *QuESTA Learning Cycle* student reading and the *Grape Explorations* and *Grape Experiment* activity sheets for each student.

- Review the questions on the *Grape Explorations* and *Grape Experiment* activity sheets.

- Post the *Six Steps to an Experiment* lesson resource at the front of the class.

- Review the *QuESTA!* lesson resource.

- If you have not already done so, post the Module Question and Unit 1 Question at the front of the classroom.

MODULE QUESTION

How does nature provide us with food?

UNIT QUESTION

What is a food scientist?

 QUESTIONING

1. Review Module and Unit Questions

Explain that in this lesson students will investigate grapes. As food scientists, students will explore ways to turn grapes into grape juice.

2. Explore Grapes

Pass out 3–4 grapes to each student. Have students share what they already know about grapes. Record their ideas on the board. Ask students to think about some ways that food scientists might investigate grapes. Brainstorm different ways to make observations about the grapes. Encourage students to break the grapes in half and to use all of their senses, including taste, to learn more about this fruit. Challenge students to discover something they did not know about grapes before. Have students record their findings on the *Grape Explorations* activity sheet.

Ask volunteers to share their observations. Accept all answers. Encourage discussion, questions, and debate among the students.

 EXPERIMENTING

3. Develop Experiment Procedure

Have students work in groups of 3–4 students to develop an experimental procedure to answer the question: *How is grape juice made from grapes?* Students in each group can record the methods and materials on their *Grape Explorations* activity sheet. Encourage students to include as much detail as possible.

4. Have Groups Share Their Methods

Have each group write its method on the board or on chart paper. Invite groups to present their methods to the class. Encourage student groups to ask questions of their classmates. Explore similarities and differences among the groups' methods. *What steps did all the groups include? What steps did only some groups include? What steps seem to be very important to turn grapes into grape juice? Do you think any steps listed are not important? Why?* Most likely, all the groups included smashing the grapes as part of their method. Investigate each group's grape-smashing method. Be sure to discuss how to handle the seeds and skins. *How would you guess the grape juice might turn out using these different mashing methods? What ideas do you have for handling the seeds and skin of the grapes?*

5. Plan Whole-Class Experimental Procedure

Consider all of the groups' experimental procedures. Then, as a whole class, develop one method to use in Lesson 3 when you will make grape juice from grapes. This is an excellent opportunity to model how to plan a complete, detailed procedure for an experiment. Write your methods on chart paper so they can be posted when you do Lesson 3. If you wish to have students record the class experiment, they can copy it into their LiFE Logs. See the *Grapes and Grape Juice* teacher note for a description of how grape juice is made.

Make a materials list and determine where you will get the supplies. You may wish to have students bring in some of the kitchen supplies that are needed. Modify methods, as necessary, based on available materials.

Create a class hypothesis for the experiment. Or, you can have the students write their own hypotheses in their LiFE Logs.

Alternative method: Instead of creating one class experiment, let each group try the process as designed. This way the class can compare results and each group can learn what works and does not work in their experimental procedure. However, this will take more materials and more time.

 SEARCHING

6. Introduce QuESTA Learning Cycle

Explain that LiFE uses the QuESTA Learning Cycle to help students understand the process of learning. *Have you ever thought about how you learn? What might be the steps involved in learning something new? Can you share with the class an example of how you learned something?*

Distribute the *QuESTA Learning Cycle* student reading. Have students read it individually or as a class. Discuss each phase and ask students to define each one using their own words. Encourage questions and discussion.

 THEORIZING

7. LiFE Logs

Have students write a paragraph that begins with: "Today I learned some new things about grapes. Here's what I learned..." Ask students to include a description of the kind of observations they made. Prompt them to describe what they learned by using each of their senses. Remind them to include any questions they still have about grapes.

QuESTA!

How students learn is as important as what they learn. The Module and Unit questions ask students to think hard by challenging them to explore, question, investigate, analyze, synthesize, and act. QuESTA is a five-phase cycle that guides students through this process. Although the phases are presented linearly, they are dynamic. Once you get acquainted with QuESTA, you and your students will flow among the phases. Here are some sample questions to help you guide your students' learning.

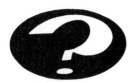

QUESTIONING

- What do I already know about the topic?
- What don't I know about the topic but would like to learn?
- What am I curious about?
- How might I find answers to my questions?
- What if…?

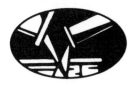

EXPERIMENTING

- How can I set up my experiment?
- What are the steps in my experiment?
- What materials do I need for my experiment?
- What do I think will happen?
- Did my experiment work as well as I thought it would? Is there anything I would like to change about it?
- What data do I have?
- What are the results of my experiment?

SEARCHING

- What can I learn from reading or talking to people?
- Where can I find out more information?
- What do scientists already know about this topic?
- How can I find out if my results are accurate?
- How can I tell the difference between a fact and an opinion?

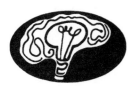

THEORIZING

- What have I learned?
- What evidence do I have to support my conclusion?
- Have my ideas changed?
- What are some different ways that I can analyze what I have learned from questioning, experimenting and searching?
- What conclusions can I draw?
- Has my thinking about this topic changed? Why or why not?

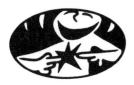

APPLYING TO LIFE

- How can I use what I have learned?
- How can I remember to think about what I have learned as I do my daily activities?
- What can I teach my family and friends?
- What new questions do I have about the topic now that I am using this new knowledge in the real world?

Six Steps to an Experiment

Step 1: Develop an experiment question. This is the question your experiment is trying to answer. To develop a question, think about what you want to learn.

Ask Yourself: What question do I want to answer with my experiment?

Step 2: Decide on a **hypothesis.** A hypothesis is a prediction, or a guess, about the results of the experiment.

Ask Yourself: What do I think will happen?

Step 3: Develop your **experimental design.** Write down the steps you will do to conduct the experiment. These are called your methods. If you are conducting an experiment to make comparisons, identify the **control group** and the **experimental group.** With the experimental group, be sure to identify the **variable** (the thing that will change). Include a list of the materials you will need for your experiment.

Ask Yourself: What are all the steps in my experiment? What materials do I need to conduct the experiment?

Step 4: Do the experiment following your methods.

Ask Yourself: Is my experiment working as planned? Does it need to be changed? How could I change it to make it better?

Step 5: Record your data in a table, a chart, or in your LiFE Log.

Ask Yourself: What are the results? How should I record my data? Should I use a chart, a graph, a table, or write a paragraph to describe my results?

Step 6: Examine your results and think about what you have learned. Use your answers to this question to make your conclusions.

Ask Yourself: What did my experiment teach me, and how can I use this?

Grapes and Grape Juice

Did you know that grapes are the most commonly grown fruit in the world? This fruit and its juice have been popular for a long time. Archaeologists have found evidence of fermented grape juice in pottery jars dated to Neolithic times, about 5400 to 5000 B.C. And even though wild grapes didn't grow in ancient Egypt, artwork on tomb walls depicts the wine-making process. Extracting juice from grapes has a long history!

What's the first thing you think of when you think about making grape juice? For most people, smashing grapes — whether with feet or food processor — is what first comes to mind. Undoubtedly, this will also be the first thing that comes to your students' minds as well. You can count on hearing some rather creative ideas for smashing the fruit! While smashing grapes is part of the process, a very important step occurs after the smashing. This is the step when the grape pulp is heated. The heating process brings out the sugar in the grapes and incorporates elements from the skins. If purple grapes are used, the juice takes on the purple color of the skin.

Grape-Juice Recipe

Most grape-juice recipes recommend mashing the grapes with a potato masher, then heating the grapes to boiling. Continue to mash the grapes during heating. After the grape pulp boils for about 3 minutes, reduce the heat and simmer for 20 minutes. The final step is straining the juice through a fine strainer or cheesecloth to remove any remaining skin fragments and seeds. If possible, try heating your grapes when your class makes grape juice. Even if you don't do it in class, perhaps you, or one of your students, could try adding the heating step at home and bringing in the juice for everyone to try. Commercial grape juice is heated at least one more time during the pasteurization process before it reaches store shelves.

Most commercial grape juice is made from Concord grapes, which have a deep purple skin but light green insides. Concord grapes are highly perishable and can be hard to find in stores. If they grow in your region, you may be able to find them in farmers' markets. Another popular variety to look for is Niagara.

Scientific Inquiry

With this lesson, LiFE introduces students to the scientific method. Your students will gain valuable experience recording and describing each step in the grape juice-making procedure.

It's important for students to understand that different kinds of investigations are used to answer different kinds of questions. Sometimes observation might be appropriate. *How does a starfish move?* Sometimes a question can be answered through research. *Are all grapes purple?* Sometimes a thought analysis can answer a question. *Could animals live if there were no plants?* Other times, a controlled experiment can be used to answer the question. *Does the amount of light affect how a plant grows?* In an experiment, scientists need to control the variables — the factors that can affect the results. For example, water, air, and temperature might also affect plant growth. To test just the effect of light, a scientist would control the other factors (water, temperature, and air).

While students are introduced to controlled experiments in this lesson, they do not conduct one until Lesson 4. You may choose to save your discussion of controls and variables until later in this unit.

Name   Date

QuESTA Learning Cycle

You have been learning science since you were born. Have you ever thought about how you learn? You will in the LiFE program!

In the LiFE program, you will use the QuESTA Learning Cycle. When you first begin to study a topic, you will question what you already know about the topic. For example, what do you already know about grapes? After you think about what you already know, you ask yourself what **questions** you still have about grapes.

How can you find answers to the questions you still have? One way is to conduct a scientific test called an **experiment.** When you conduct an experiment, you may make new discoveries or develop new ideas as you try to find answers to your questions. You may also **search** for more information by reading or talking to people.

What do you do with all of this new information you've learned from questioning, doing experiments, and searching? You can use it to develop new **theories,** or explanations of how things work.

You may be asking yourself how you can use what you have learned. Try using it in your daily life and sharing it with your family. For example, the next time you have a glass of grape juice, think about how it was made. You may even want to teach your family and friends what you've learned. When you do this, you'll be **applying to life** what you have learned.

Once you start applying what you learned, you may find you have more questions. This starts the learning cycle all over again.

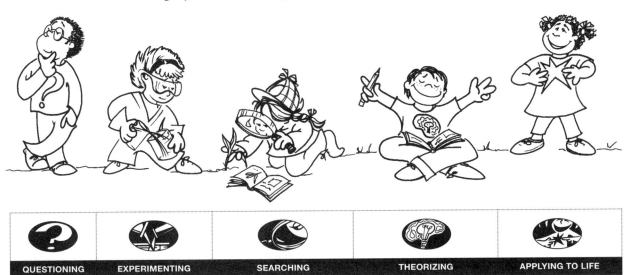

| QUESTIONING | EXPERIMENTING | SEARCHING | THEORIZING | APPLYING TO LIFE |

Name

Date

Grape Explorations

Answer the following questions.

1. What do you already know about grapes?

_____

_____

_____

_____

_____

2. Look at your grapes very closely and record some of your new observations.

_____

_____

_____

_____

_____

_____

_____

(continued on next page)

Name		Date

Grape Explorations

3. Make a drawing of the grape and what you observe.

4. Based on what you already know about grapes and what you have just learned from your observations, write down some ideas about how you think grapes are turned into grape juice.

_____

_____

_____

_____

_____

_____

BECOMING FOOD SCIENTISTS :: PLANTS :: FOOD WEBS :: AGRICULTURE :: MAKING CHOICES

Name   Date

Grape Experiment

Answer the following questions.

Research Question: *How can we make grape juice from grapes?*

1. Working with your group, list all of the steps that are needed to make grape juice from grapes. Try to include every step from start to finish. These are called your methods.

_____

_____

_____

_____

_____

_____

_____

_____

_____

_____

_____

(continued on next page)

Name   Date

Grape Experiment

2. List everything you will need for your grape juice-making procedure. Think through the entire process and try not to leave anything out.

_____

_____

_____

_____

_____

_____

3. What do you think your results will be?

_____

_____

_____

_____

_____

_____

Growing Food
©2007 Teachers College Columbia University

BECOMING FOOD SCIENTISTS : PLANTS : FOOD WEBS : AGRICULTURE : MAKING CHOICES

Making Grape Juice

AIM

To continue to learn about grapes and QuESTA through making grape juice and synthesizing new ideas about grapes.

SCIENTIFIC PROCESSES

- **experiment, gather data, infer, theorize, apply**

OBJECTIVES

Students will be able to:

- **describe their experiences of making grape juice from grapes;**

- **develop theories on how commercial grape juice is made, based on what they have learned about grapes;**

- **express in writing in their LiFE Logs what it will be like to learn using QuESTA.**

OVERVIEW

Students learn more about the QuESTA Learning Cycle. They continue with the Experimenting phase by conducting their class experiment for making grape juice, doing the experiment and variations on it as many times as they can. After the experiment they move to the Theorizing phase through speculating on how store-bought grape juice is made. They speculate on how much effort it took to make a small amount of juice and come up with ideas about how factories might make very large amounts of grape juice. This gives them the opportunity to process what they have learned in order to synthesize new knowledge constructs, something they will do through-out the LiFE Curriculum Series. Finally, they Apply the lesson to life by discussing what they will think, feel, and do differently in the future, based on what they have learned about grapes and grape juice.

MATERIALS

For the class:
- 3 bunches of grapes

- Chart paper with experiment recorded (from Lesson 2)

- Materials as listed for class experiment (from Lesson 2)

For each student:
- *Turning Grapes into Juice* activity sheet

- *Grape Juice Theories* activity sheet

- *Applying What I Have Learned* activity sheet

- LiFE Log

PROCEDURE

Before You Begin:

- Complete any setup needed for your experiment.

- Post the experiment recorded on chart paper in Lesson 2.

- Make enough copies of the *Turning Grapes into Juice, Grape Juice Theories,* and *Applying What I Have Learned* activity sheets for each student.

- If you have not already done so, post the Module Question and Unit 1 Question at the front of the classroom.

MODULE QUESTION

How does nature provide us with food?

UNIT QUESTION

What is a food scientist?

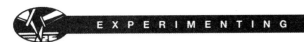

1. Review Module and Unit Questions

Explain that in this lesson the class is going to conduct an experiment. Conducting experiments is one way that food scientists learn more about food.

2. Conduct Grape Juice Experiment

As the experiment is being done, help the students see how you are following the methods just as they were written up in the last session. If you have the supplies and the time, conduct the experiment a second time to compare with the results from the first time. You may do the experiment in the exact same way or make modifications based on what you learned the first time. Explain to the students that scientists often do experiments more than once to determine if their results come out the same each time. If the results are different, scientists carefully look over what they did to determine why.

3. Record Results

Have students describe the results of the experiment on the *Turning Grapes into Juice* activity sheet. Review the questions on the activity sheet with students. Check for understanding. Have students answer the questions.

4. Develop Grape Juice Theories

From what you learned in your experiment, how do you think the grape juice you buy in the store is made? Discuss as a whole class, then have students write their answers on the *Grape Juice Theories* activity sheet.

Encourage students to think about the factories that make grape juice in very large quantities. *How might what happens in a factory be similar to what we did in class? How might it be different? What do you think factories do with the seeds and skins of the grapes? How might the equipment used in a factory be like the equipment we used in class? How might it be different?* Use the teacher note in Lesson 2 to guide you through this discussion.

Remind students that the theorizing phase of QuESTA is particularly important. It is their opportunity to put together everything they have learned and to gain new knowledge about what they are studying that they will be able to use now and in the future.

5. Share Written Answers

Encourage questions, discussion, and debate among the students. Continue the conversation until you feel most students have developed a new understanding about making grape juice.

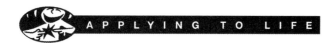
6. Discuss Applications

Ask students to describe how their thoughts and actions related to grapes and grape juice have changed as a result of this lesson. Have students complete the *Applying What I Have Learned* activity sheet.

Explain that in this final phase of the learning cycle, students will think about how they will apply what they learned to their daily decisions.

7. LiFE Logs

Have students define in their own words the five phases of QuESTA (Questioning, Experimenting, Searching, Theorizing, and Applying to Life) and describe what they think it will be like to learn using the QuESTA Learning Cycle.

Name   Date

Turning Grapes into Juice

Use these questions to help you describe the results of your experiment.

1. Does what you made look like grape juice?

_____

_____

_____

2. How is the juice you made similar to grape juice you have had before? How is it different?

_____

_____

_____

_____

3. Is the juice thick or thin? What is the texture?

_____

_____

_____

(continued on next page)

Name   Date

Turning Grapes into Juice

4. Does the juice have skin or seeds in it?

_____

_____

_____

_____

5. How does it smell? How does it taste?

_____

_____

_____

_____

6. Compare your results with your hypothesis. What was similar? What was different?

_____

_____

_____

_____

(continued on next page)

Growing Food
©2007 Teachers College Columbia University

Name	Date

Turning Grapes into Juice

7. What worked about your experiment? Why?

_____

_____

_____

_____

8. What didn't work about your experiment? Why?

_____

_____

_____

_____

9. What would you do differently next time? Why?

_____

_____

_____

_____

BECOMING FOOD SCIENTISTS : PLANTS : FOOD WEBS : AGRICULTURE : MAKING CHOICES

Name   Date

Grape Juice Theories

Now that you have made grape juice, you're ready to start developing some theories about how the grape juice you buy in the store is made. Remember how you made grape juice in class. To develop your theories, you will need to think about what you have learned, what evidence you have to support your theory, and how your ideas about grape juice may have changed. Maybe you have some new, or different, ideas about grape juice. Think about what you know about grapes and grape juice. Now think about what you learned by making the juice.

1. How do you think the grape juice you buy in the store is made?

_____

_____

_____

_____

_____

_____

_____

_____

(continued on next page)

Name   Date

Grape Juice Theories

2. What evidence do you have for your ideas?

_____

_____

_____

_____

_____

3. How have your ideas changed?

_____

_____

_____

_____

_____

Name	Date

Applying What I Have Learned

Now that you've completed your experiment and developed theories about grape juice, it's time to think about how you can use what you have learned in your life. Maybe you want to teach other people how to make grape juice. Perhaps you will think about the kind of grapes that were used to make the juice you drink, where the juice was made, and how it was made. Maybe you'll discover that as you think about making grape juice, you have even more questions that you'd like to investigate. There are no right or wrong answers. This is a time for you to put into action what you have learned in this lesson.

1. How will you use what you learned about grapes and grape juice in the future?

_____

_____

_____

_____

_____

_____

_____

_____

(continued on next page)

LESSON 3: MAKING GRAPE JUICE

Name	Date

Applying What I Have Learned

2. Based on what you have learned about making grape juice in class, do you have any new questions about the grape juice you buy in the store?

_____

_____

_____

_____

_____

_____

3. How can you apply what you have learned to your daily life? Is there anything that you will do differently?

_____

_____

_____

_____

_____

_____

Growing Food
©2007 Teachers College Columbia University

BECOMING FOOD SCIENTISTS : PLANTS : FOOD WEBS : AGRICULTURE : MAKING CHOICES

Pre-Assessment

AIM

To assess what we already know about how nature provides us with food.

SCIENTIFIC PROCESSES

- **question, assess knowledge, predict**

OBJECTIVES

Students will be able to:

- **express in a picture and in writing how nature provides us with food;**

- **appreciate how the Module and Unit questions will guide everything they learn in the module;**

- **predict what will happen to plant leaves when they are covered.**

OVERVIEW

Students are reintroduced to the Module Question and reminded that this question frames everything they learn in this module. Students are also introduced to the Unit 2, 3, 4, and 5 questions to demonstrate that Unit Questions will help them understand the Module Question. Students draw a detailed picture that represents their ideas about the Module Question. This activity helps students realize what they already know and prompts them to wonder what they will learn. Then, using their picture as a guide, students write a paragraph in their LiFE Logs describing how nature provides us with food. Reviewing this paragraph as they work through the module will allow students to track what they have learned. In this lesson, students also set up experiments using houseplants. These experiments are a brief introduction to the complex process of photosynthesis.

MATERIALS

For the teacher:
- *Blocking the Light* experiment sheet
- *Blocking the Stomata* experiment sheet
- *Assessing What Your Students Already Know* teacher note

For the class:
- Chart paper
- Markers
- 2 houseplants (geraniums work well)
- Aluminum foil

- 4 paper clips
- 2 pebbles
- 2 clear plastic bags
- Scissors
- Petroleum jelly
- Tape or twist ties

For each student:
- 1 large white index card
- Markers or crayons
- LiFE Log
- *Plant Leaf Experiment Predictions* activity sheet

PROCEDURE

Before You Begin:

- Gather the materials for the plant leaf experiment.

- Review the *Blocking the Light* and *Blocking the Stomata* experiment sheets.

- Review the *Assessing What Your Students Already Know* teacher note.

- If you have not already done so, post the Module Question and the Unit 1 Question at the front of the classroom.

MODULE QUESTION

How does nature provide us with food?

UNIT QUESTION

What is a food scientist?

 QUESTIONING

1. Reintroduce Module Question

Remind students of the Module Question. Post the lesson resource version of this question. Engage students in a class discussion. Point out that the Module Question frames everything they will do throughout this module. To become familiar with studying food and how LiFE works, we investigated the Unit 1 Question. To better understand how nature provides us with food, we will investigate four more Unit Questions: Unit 2: *If there were no plants, would humans have food?* Unit 3: *How do components in nature interact with each other?* Unit 4: *How do we interact with nature to meet our food needs?* And Unit 5: *How can we use the science we learned to make food and agriculture choices?* Post these questions along with the Module Question.

Elicit students' ideas about how nature provides us with food. Record these ideas on chart paper or on the board. The list may include: plants, vegetables, cows, other animals, sun, rain, everything in nature, fruit, chickens, farms, farmers, crops, and so forth. Accept all answers.

2. Create a Picture

Ask students to draw a picture on an index card that represents how nature provides us with food. Encourage the use of diagrams, words, and arrows.

3. Share Pictures

After students have finished drawing, invite them to share their work with the class. Encourage support of each other, questions, and comments during this sharing. Display the drawings in your classroom and keep them out throughout the time you work on the module. Some teachers have made the index cards into a "quilt" and displayed it on a bulletin board. Others have turned the cards into a book. What's important is making certain the drawings are prominently displayed throughout the module.

4. LiFE Logs

Have students write an answer to the Module Question. They can use their picture as a guide.

Through recording what they already know about this question, students will be able to assess how their thinking changes as they go through the module lessons. This process of assessing their own understanding and knowledge can be a stimulating academic challenge. Be sure to spend time discussing this with students and brainstorming ideas they have in order to track their learning. With each lesson, be sure to provide time for students to share what they have learned with their classmates.

5. Assign Homework

Have students write two questions they have about food production in their LiFE Logs.

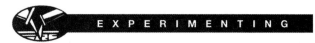

EXPERIMENTING

6. Experiment Setup

Explain that to begin to learn about plants, the class is going to do experiments to see what happens to plant leaves when they are blocked from the light. In the first experiment, part of a leaf is covered with aluminum foil. In the second experiment, the bottom of one leaf is coated with petroleum jelly and a plastic bag is wrapped around the leaf. Another leaf on the same plant is wrapped in a plastic bag but is not coated with petroleum jelly. Both plants are set out in a sunny location. Refer to the *Blocking the Light* and *Blocking the Stomata* experiment sheets to set up these experiments. After the experiments are set up, have students complete the *Plant Leaf Experiment Predictions* activity sheet. Invite some students to share their answers. Save the experiment sheets and activity sheets. You will refer to them during Lesson 5 as students complete their plant leaf investigations.

Blocking the Light

Students will observe what happens when aluminum foil covers part of a plant leaf and the plant is placed in a sunny location.

Setup

Cut several pieces of aluminum foil that are larger than the plant leaves.

Procedure

1. Cut shapes out of the aluminum foil to cover part of a few leaves. Be sure the shapes are large enough to cover at least half of the surface of the leaf.

2. Attach the aluminum foil shapes to a few leaves using paper clips.

3. Put the plant in a sunny location.

4. Be sure to water the plant throughout the experiment.

5. Leave the plant for several days before removing the foil covers.

Questions

1. What will happen when aluminum foil covers the plant's leaves? Why do you think this will happen?

2. What is blocked from reaching the leaves?

3. Why is sunlight important to plants?

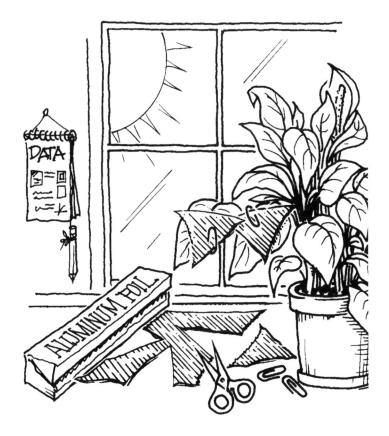

Blocking the Stomata

In this experiment, one plant leaf is coated with petroleum jelly and another is not. Both leaves are covered with plastic bags that are weighted with small pebbles. Students observe what happens after the plant leaves are left for at least one day.

Setup

Use a houseplant with a large leaf surface or, if you can do this outside, use the leaves on a tree. You may want to make a sign that indicates an experiment is in progress.

Procedure

1. Coat the underside of a leaf with petroleum jelly.

2. Place one of the plastic bags over the leaf with the petroleum jelly coating. Put a pebble in the bag near the tip of the leaf.

3. Secure the plastic at the top of the leaf with tape or a twist tie. Make it snug, but not tight enough to cause damage to the stem.

4. Place the other plastic bag over a leaf that does not have the petroleum jelly coating. Put a pebble in the bag near the tip of the leaf.

5. Secure the plastic at the top of the leaf with tape or a twist tie. Make it snug, but not tight enough to cause damage to the stem.

6. Put the plant in a sunny location and wait at least one day.

7. Be sure to water the plant throughout the experiment.

Questions

1. What is located on the underside of a leaf that is blocked by the petroleum jelly?

2. What do you think will happen to a leaf that has petroleum jelly on the bottom?

3. What do you think will happen to the leaf that does not have the petroleum jelly coating but is covered by a plastic bag?

4. Do you notice any changes in the plastic bags? If so, in which one, or is it in both? What do you observe? Why do you think this happened?

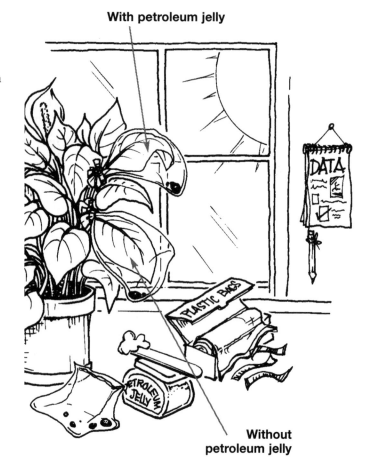

With petroleum jelly

Without petroleum jelly

Assessing What Your Students Already Know

The first unit of this module, *Becoming Food Scientists,* familiarized students with studying food, inquiry-based science, and the phases of the QuESTA Learning Cycle. Units 2–5 are about growing food. This lesson is an authentic assessment that allows your students to record their current thinking about the Module Question and to track how their thinking changes as they complete the lessons in this module. We have found that when students fully understand and explore the Module Question at the beginning of the module, they are more fully engaged throughout the entire module. Please make it clear to students that what they draw in their picture and what they write in their LiFE Logs offers an understanding of what they know right now. Make it a fun challenge for students to really think through what they know right now. By doing a good job with this today, they can chart what they learn throughout the module, since they will draw another picture and write an answer to the Module Question again in Lesson 20 at the end of the module. This lesson also offers an opportunity to set up how each of the unit questions builds to a greater understanding of the Module Question.

BECOMING FOOD SCIENTISTS : PLANTS : FOOD WEBS : AGRICULTURE : MAKING CHOICES

Name	Date

Plant Leaf Experiment Predictions

1. What does the aluminum foil cover do to the leaves?

_____

_____

_____

2. What do you think will happen to the part of the leaf that is under the aluminum foil? Why do you think this will happen?

_____

_____

_____

_____

_____

3. Why is sunlight important to plants?

_____

_____

_____

_____

(continued on next page)

LESSON 4: PRE-ASSESSMENT

Name	Date

Plant Leaf Experiment Predictions

4. What are we blocking by coating the underside of a leaf with petroleum jelly?

_____

_____

_____

_____

5. What do you think will happen to the leaves with the plastic bags covering them? Will anything collect in the plastic?

_____

_____

_____

_____

_____

_____

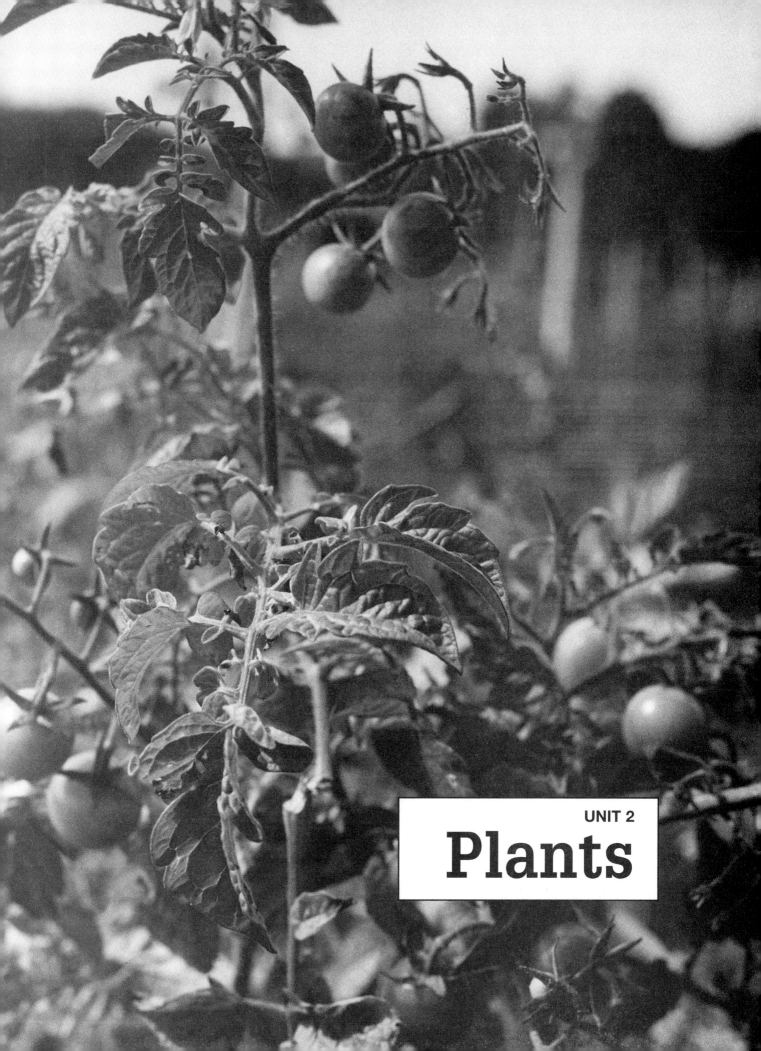

UNIT 2
Plants

LESSON 5

The Producers

AIM

To investigate how plants get energy.

SCIENTIFIC PROCESSES

question, investigate, gather data, build theories

OBJECTIVES

Students will be able to:

- **explain what happens when plant leaves are not exposed to sunlight;**

- **describe how plants lose water into the air;**

- **further their understanding of the structure and function of plant leaves;**

- **discuss the importance of the sun for plants.**

OVERVIEW

In this lesson students continue the investigations of green plants that they began in Lesson 4. Students focus their investigations on the structure and function of plants and energy transformation as they begin to explore the question for this unit: *If there were no plants, would humans have food?* Students collect the data from the plant experiments and analyze their results. These experiments are students' first experiences with experimental design in the LiFE program. We encourage you to review with students *Six Steps to an Experiment* (p. 38). After you have reviewed the experimental design and students' predictions from Lesson 4, students gather data, record it in their LiFE Logs, and then discuss the data as a class, including ways to display the data and describe the results. With this lesson students begin in earnest their exploration of the Module Question: *How does nature provide us with food?*

MATERIALS

For the teacher:
- *Blocking the Light* experiment sheet (p. 59)
- *Blocking the Stomata* experiment sheet (p. 60)
- *Six Steps to an Experiment* lesson resource (p. 38)
- *Plant Leaf Theories* sample conversation
- Chart paper
- Markers
- (Optional) Overhead projector
- (Optional) Overhead transparency film

For the class:
- Plants from the experiments in Lesson 4

For each student:
- *Plant Leaf Experiment Predictions* activity sheet (pp. 62–63)
- *Plant Experiment Theories* activity sheet
- *What Plants Need to Grow* student reading
- LiFE Log

PROCEDURE

Before You Begin:

- If you have not already done so, complete the experiment set up in Lesson 4.

- Review the questions on the **Blocking the Light** and **Blocking the Stomata** experiment sheets.

- Review the **Six Steps to an Experiment** lesson resource. (Optional) Make an overhead transparency of this resource. If you choose not to make an overhead transparency, you may wish to transfer the text to chart paper to post at the front of the class.

- Make a copy of the **What Plants Need to Grow** reading and the **Plant Experiment Theories** activity sheet for each student.

- If you have not already done so, post the Module Question and Unit 2 Question at the front of the classroom.

MODULE QUESTION

How does nature provide us with food?

UNIT QUESTION

If there were no plants, would humans have food?

 QUESTIONING

1. Review Student Understanding of Plants

Elicit from students their ideas about the difference between plants and animals. Accept all answers and record them on chart paper. If students have not already included the fact that plants can make their own food and animals cannot, introduce this idea. Create a concept map with the words "green plants" in the middle. Encourage students to present any thoughts and ideas they have about plants. Accept all answers and add them to the concept map.

2. Introduce the Unit 2 Question

Remind students that in their **Growing Food** studies, they have been investigating the Module Question. In Unit 2, the class will be investigating green plants and their connection to the food humans eat. You may wish to post the questions at the front of the classroom and invite volunteers to read them out loud to the class.

 EXPERIMENTING

3. Experimental Design

Ask students to take out their completed **Plant Leaf Experiment Predictions** activity sheet from Lesson 4. Have students work in pairs as you review the experiments. Give them time to discuss the experimental design as well as their predictions. Pick two volunteers to be the food scientists. Each student food scientist will explain one of the two plant leaf experiments. Use the overhead transparency or chart paper of **Six Steps to an Experiment** to guide the students' discussion. *What question were we trying to answer with the experiment that used the aluminum foil? What was the hypothesis? What did you predict would happen? What question were we trying to answer with the experiment that used the petroleum jelly? What was the hypothesis? What did you predict would happen?*

Be sure to spend time discussing the control group, the experimental group, and the variable. *In the experiment with the aluminum foil, what was the variable?* (The amount of light the leaf receives.) *What was done with the experimental leaf to block exposure to light?* (It was covered with foil.) *What was done to the control leaves?* (Nothing, so they got the usual amount of light.) *In the experiment with the petroleum jelly, what was the variable?* (Petroleum jelly on the bottom surface of the leaf. The petroleum jelly blocks gases from going in or out of the stomata that are on the bottom of the leaf.) *What was done to the experimental leaf?* (The bottom surface was covered with petroleum jelly and the leaf was covered with a plastic bag.) *What was done to the control leaf?* (It was covered with a plastic bag.) End this discussion at Step 4.

4. Gather Data

Divide the class in half. Have one half gather and analyze the data for the **Blocking the Light** experiment while the other half gathers and analyzes the data for the **Blocking the Stomata** experiment. You may wish to have students work in small groups and take turns examining the experiments and gathering the data. Have students work in their small groups to discuss different ways to display their data. Let them choose one way and prepare the data to share with the class. *What are you comparing? What do you need to label or identify? Would a graph or a table help you organize your data? Are there other ways you want to organize your results?*

 THEORIZING

5. Discuss Results

Invite representatives from the **Blocking the Light** group of students and the **Blocking the Stomata** group of students to present their data. *What does your data show? Were you surprised by these results? Did the experiments work as*

planned? Would you change anything? Have students look at the results and think about what they have learned.

6. Build Theories

Distribute the **Plant Experiment Theories** activity sheet to each student. Give students a few moments to review the questions and record their answers. Remind them to cite the evidence they are using to draw their conclusions. Encourage a whole-class discussion of the conclusions that can be drawn based on the evidence from the two experiments.

7. LiFE Logs

Have students answer the questions: *Why is the sun so important for plants?* and *What new things have I learned about plants?* Remind students to cite the evidence that supports their conclusion. Encourage them to include new questions they may have as a result of doing these experiments.

8. Homework

Give each student a copy of the **What Plants Need to Grow** student reading to read after they complete this lesson.

Plant Leaf Theories

This sample conversation in the *Theorizing* phase of the QuESTA cycle will help you guide your students through a conversation that will enable them to construct new knowledge. As you engage students in your own conversation, encourage them to debate the interpretation of the results of their experiment, to explain their own theories about what they learned, and to recognize how they might use this new knowledge in their daily lives. This is a guide. Feel free to adjust your questioning to the needs of your class.

MR. S: Let's think about the results of our two plant experiments. *Why do you think the leaf that was covered with foil looks different from the leaves that weren't covered?*

JACK: Once I was in the park and I picked up a large stone that was on top of the grass. Underneath the stone, the grass wasn't green. It was almost white. My mom said the stone blocked the light so the grass couldn't turn green. Maybe the stone and the foil both block light.

MR. S: That's an interesting observation. *What effect do you think sunlight has on a plant?*

ANNA: My grandmother had a plant in her apartment that died. She told me it didn't get enough light. Maybe plants need light to live.

MR. S: Good thinking. So far our evidence tells us that when sunlight is blocked, plant leaves do not turn green, and we have evidence that plants that don't get enough light die. *Based on this evidence, what conclusion can we make about the importance of sunlight to plants?*

ANNA: Plants need sunlight to live.

MR. S: Your reasoning is very good. *Now, what can we learn about leaves from our other experiment with the petroleum jelly? What were your results and what do they tell you?*

JACK: One plastic bag had water drops in it and the one over the leaf with the petroleum jelly

didn't have any water. It makes me wonder where the water came from. Maybe it's hot inside the bag. When I run around and get hot, I sweat. Maybe one of the plants is sweating. Maybe the plant leaf is like my skin and has tiny holes in it that the water comes through, like the pores in my skin.

MR. S: That's an interesting comparison to sweating, Jack. *What about the leaf with the petroleum jelly? Does that tell us anything?*

JACK: When I swim, I put petroleum jelly on my swim goggles so they don't leak. It keeps the water out. Maybe it can also keep the water in the leaf since we didn't see any water in that plastic bag.

MR. S: Based on what we've learned, I have some new questions. *Where do you think the water comes from? Do you think anything can enter the leaves the same way the water goes out?* Now, let's turn to our LiFE Logs and write about what we've learned and new questions that we have.

BECOMING FOOD SCIENTISTS : PLANTS : FOOD WEBS : AGRICULTURE : MAKING CHOICES

Name	Date

Plant Experiment Theories

Blocking the Light

1. What conclusions can you draw from the experiment?

_____

_____

_____

2. How might you confirm the importance of light to plants?

_____

_____

_____

Blocking the Stomata

1. What conclusions can you draw from the experiment?

_____

_____

_____

2. What evidence do you have?

_____

_____

_____

LESSON 5: THE PRODUCERS

Growing Food
©2007 Teachers College Columbia University

Name	Date

What Plants Need to Grow

How are animals and green plants different? One big difference is that animals can eat food. Plants cannot. Green plants, like this tomato plant, make their own food. They are called **producers** — they produce their own food using light energy, water, and carbon dioxide to make sugars, their food. Plants get light energy from the sun, water from the soil, and carbon dioxide from the air.

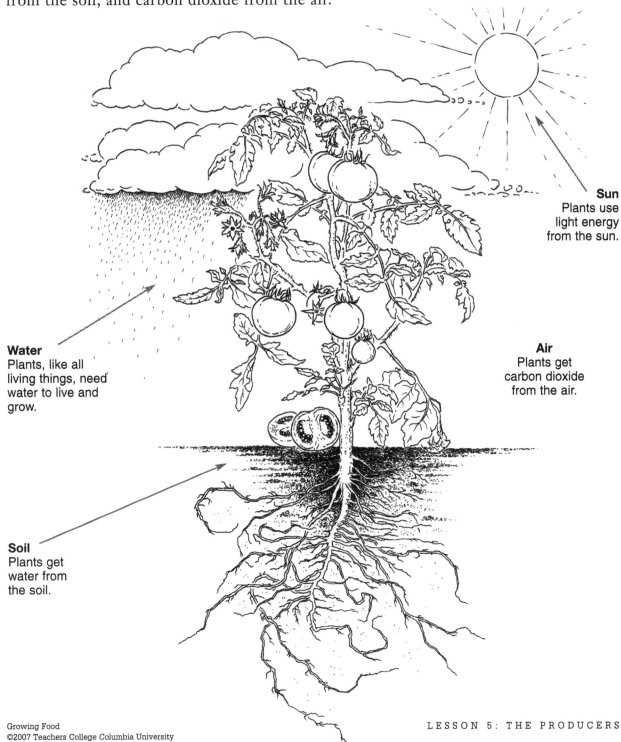

Sun
Plants use light energy from the sun.

Water
Plants, like all living things, need water to live and grow.

Air
Plants get carbon dioxide from the air.

Soil
Plants get water from the soil.

Celebrating Plant Parts

AIM

To further student understanding of plants and to enjoy eating a variety of plant parts.

SCIENTIFIC PROCESSES

observe, experiment, apply

OBJECTIVES

Students will be able to:

- **identify the structure and function of plant parts;**
- **identify edible plant parts;**
- **describe food preparation procedures for safety, sanitation, and enjoyment;**
- **appreciate the wide array of foods that we can get from plants.**

OVERVIEW

In this lesson students continue their exploration of plants. They learn more about the structure and function of roots, stems, leaves, flowers, fruit, and seeds. This lesson may be challenging for some of your students. They are asked to think about plants as botanists do. In the process, students may discover that the word "vegetable" is not a botanical term and what they thought was a vegetable is botanically a fruit. Challenge your students to think like botanists for part of this lesson. When they put on their chefs' hats, they will be back in the world of "vegetables!" To celebrate what they have learned, the class makes a salad. We hope this lesson deepens your students' appreciation of the important role plants play in our lives and inspires students to consume more foods from plants. We encourage you to use the salad-making activity as an opportunity to reinforce the fact that we eat, and get energy from, all different parts of plants.

MATERIALS

For the teacher:
- *Salad Grocery List* lesson resource
- *Kitchen Supplies and Equipment* lesson resource
- *Cooking Tips* lesson resource
- *Classroom Salad* recipe
- *Classroom Salad Dressing* recipe

For the class:
- (Optional) Hand towels
- Materials from the *Salad Grocery List* and *Kitchen Supplies and Equipment* lesson resources.

For each student:
- *Tomatoes: From Roots to Seeds* student reading
- *Roots* student reading
- *Stems* student reading
- *Leaves* student reading
- *Flowers* student reading
- *Fruit* student reading
- *Seeds* student reading
- *Plant Parts We Eat* activity sheet
- *Take-Home Salad* recipe
- LiFE Logs

PROCEDURE

Before You Begin:

- Make a copy of the *Tomatoes: From Roots to Seeds* reading for each student and read in literacy time before conducting this lesson.

- Make copies of the *Roots, Stems, Leaves, Flowers, Fruit* and *Seeds* readings for each student or for small groups of students. See procedure below.

- Make copies of the *Take-Home Salad* recipe and *Plant Parts We Eat* activity sheet for each student.

- Review the *Salad Grocery List, Classroom Salad* recipe, and *Classroom Salad Dressing* recipe. Purchase the ingredients for the class salad and salad dressing.

- Copy the *Cooking Tips* lesson resource onto chart paper and post it in front of the class to review with students.

- Review the *Kitchen Supplies and Equipment* and *Cooking Tips* lesson resources and gather together any materials you may need for this project.

- Make an overhead transparency of the *Classroom Salad* recipe or make enough copies of it to distribute to student groups.

- Have students wash their hands just before you begin this lesson.

- If you have not already done so, post the Module Question and Unit 2 Question at the front of the classroom.

MODULE QUESTION

How does nature provide us with food?

UNIT QUESTION

If there were no plants, would humans have food?

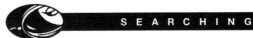

SEARCHING

1. Review Plant Parts

If you have not already read *Tomatoes: From Roots to Seeds*, read it as a class before going on with this lesson. Hold a brief discussion and invite students to discuss new information they learned about plants. Ask if they still have questions or have new questions about plant parts.

2. Review Module and Unit Questions

Remind students of the Module Question and that the question for Unit 2 explores the connection between plants and the food humans eat. Tell students they will celebrate the diversity of plants in our diet by making and eating a salad.

3. Read Student Readings about Plant Parts

Have students work in six small groups. Assign each group one plant part to read about. Have students read about their plant part and study the drawing. After they have finished reading, give students several minutes to discuss what they have learned with their group members. Invite a volunteer from each group to present what the group learned about their plant part. You may wish to post this information on chart paper at the front of the room.

4. Look at Plant Drawings

Have students look at the drawings of the carrot, asparagus, lettuce, broccoli, tomato, and sunflower plants and read the information about each of these plant parts. Point out that all the plants have roots, stems, and leaves, but only some have flowers, fruits, and seeds. Explain that for each of these plants we typically eat only one part. For the carrots, tomato, and sunflower seeds, we choose to eat the part of the plant where the most energy gets stored. *Why do we choose to eat different parts of different plants? How do you think people came to these decisions? Do you know of any plants that are completely edible?* (Beets and turnips are two examples.)

5. Observe Salad Ingredients

Have students look at the carrots, celery, lettuce, broccoli, tomatoes, and sunflower seeds. Walk around the room with each ingredient so all can see. Point out that the recipe substitutes celery for asparagus. Explain to students that celery is not a stem, it is the petiole and joins the celery leaves to the stem. Have students compare the actual ingredients to the plant-part drawings. Invite them to share what they notice. *What do farmers do to take care of these plants? Does looking at these foods make it clear that each one is a different part of the plant?*

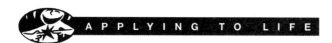 APPLYING TO LIFE

6. Establish Safe Cooking Practices

Review the *Cooking Tips* lesson resource and ask students to make additional suggestions.

7. Review the Recipe

Clarify what students will be doing with each salad ingredient (carrots: cutting the prepared carrot sticks into slices; celery: cutting the stalks into slices; lettuce: tearing the leaves into bite-sized pieces; tomatoes: cutting into bite-sized pieces; broccoli: cutting florets into bite-sized pieces). You may wish to demonstrate cutting and tearing techniques.

8. Prepare the Salad

If students have not already done so, have them wash their hands. Choose one of the following two methods for preparing the salad.

Method 1: Divide the class into 3–5 groups. Give each group some carrots, celery, lettuce, broccoli, and tomatoes to cut. This method gives all students an opportunity to prepare all the vegetables. It makes students feel more involved in the whole salad-making process. Essentially, each group makes its own salad.

Method 2: Divide the class into five groups. Give each group one vegetable to prepare. This method is easier to organize. With this method, be sure to give the lettuce group the largest bowl.

After you are certain students understand what they will be doing with the vegetables, pass out the plates and plastic knives.

As students are preparing the vegetables, make the dressing using the *Classroom Salad Dressing* recipe. You can have the first group that finishes prepare the dressing or you can invite one student from each group to make the dressing in another part of the room.

9. Put Salad Together

Once all the vegetables are prepared, bring the whole class back together. If you are using Method 1, add some sunflower seeds to each group's salad and toss well. If you are using Method 2, mix the vegetables together in the large bowl, add sunflower seeds, and toss well. If students are tossing the salad, be sure they toss it gently.

10. Cleanup

During the cleanup, make students aware that they are transforming the space where they prepared their salad into a place where they can relax and enjoy eating their salad. The cleanup can include: stacking up their cutting plates (you may want to save them to use as bedding in the compost bin in Lesson 10), washing all the plastic knives (save them for a future lesson), collecting all vegetable scraps (for the compost bin in Lesson 10) or disposing of scraps in the appropriate way for your school, wiping off all tables, picking up anything on the floor, and sweeping if necessary.

11. Eat and Enjoy

Pass out clean plates and forks. Please make sure you have enough time for the students to relax and eat. Remember to eat with your students and encourage any other adults who are in the room to join you. While students are getting ready to eat, walk around and offer dressing for their salads. After everyone finishes eating, stack the plates, wash the forks, and rinse any leftover salad if you are saving it for compost.

12. LiFE Logs

Have students write a poem or short paragraph that describes something they enjoyed and learned while making and eating the salad today.

13. Assign Homework

For homework, students will fill in the table on the *Plant Parts We Eat* activity sheet. Explain to students that it may be easier to come up with some plant parts than others. Remind students that the purpose of this activity is to help them appreciate the wide variety of foods we eat that come from plants. Distribute the *Take-Home Salad* recipe and encourage students to prepare this salad with their families.

Salad Grocery List

Now that students have learned about the structure and function of plant parts, it's time to celebrate! As a class, you will make a salad out of ingredients that demonstrate the diversity of plants and plant parts that we enjoy in our daily lives. Cooking and eating healthful food is an important part of the LiFE Curriculum Series. This salad is one of several cooking and eating experiences in the LiFE modules.

This salad recipe includes carrots, celery, broccoli, lettuce, tomatoes, and sunflower seeds. Eating plants provides us with energy, minerals, vitamins, and other nutrients. Be sure to make copies of the take-home version of this recipe so students can share it with their families. Remind them that eating a wide variety of plants each day promotes health.

SHOPPING LIST

Salad Ingredients
1 head lettuce, romaine or other dark green lettuce
1 bag mixed salad greens
7 carrots (6 for the salad and 1 for students to observe)
1 bunch celery
1 bunch of broccoli
1 pint cherry tomatoes or 7 larger tomatoes
8 ounces ready-to-eat sunflower seeds

Salad Dressing Ingredients
Olive oil
Red wine vinegar
Honey
Dijon mustard
2 shallots
2 cloves garlic
Salt and pepper

Kitchen Supplies and Equipment

You will need the following kitchen supplies and equipment to prepare the *Classroom Salad* recipe with your students.

SUPPLIES

For each student:
1 paper plate for chopping vegetables
1 paper plate to hold the serving of salad
1 plastic knife
1 plastic fork
1 napkin

Note: Use basic white paper plates with no wax or dyes if you want to save them to add to your compost box. Wash the plastic knives and forks and save to use again.

COOKING EQUIPMENT

For the teacher:
1 sharp knife for chopping
1 vegetable peeler
1 cutting board
1 spoon for serving salad dressing
2 large spoons to toss and serve salad
1 whisk

For the class:
1 bowl to mix salad dressing
1–2 large bowls to hold the salad
1 colander for rinsing vegetables

For each group of 4–6 students:
Method 1: 5–6 small bowls to hold chopped vegetables
Method 2: 1 medium bowl

Cooking Tips

Cooking with others is fun, especially if you follow these simple tips. They are not hard and will help you keep your cooking adventures safe, healthy, and enjoyable for everyone. *Bon appétit!*

Sanitation

1. Wash your hands before you begin cooking. After you have washed your hands, be sure you do not touch anything except the cooking materials. If you do, wash your hands again.

2. Try to keep food from falling on the floor. If food does fall on the floor, be sure to throw it away.

3. If you feel a cough or a sneeze coming, turn away from the food and cover your mouth. Be sure to wash your hands after coughing or sneezing.

4. Wash your hands again if you:
- scratch your head
- wipe your nose
- touch the floor
- touch anything that might make your hands dirty.

Safety

1. Be careful with all knives. Even plastic knives can hurt people.

2. Walk, do not run, jump, or skip in the classroom.

3. When you pass materials to others, do it with dignity and respect.

Making Cooking Enjoyable for All

1. Treat everyone with respect.

2. When it comes time to eat, if you don't like something, politely say, "No thank you." Please don't say it is "gross" or "nasty." Remember, you worked together as a class to prepare this food. Others want to enjoy it.

3. It's okay to talk quietly with your cooking partners. But when an adult calls for your attention, please stop talking and listen.

4. Be sure to compliment each other on a job well done.

Becoming Food Scientists :: PLANTS :: Food Webs :: Agriculture :: Making Choices

Classroom Salad

Serves 25 small portions

INGREDIENTS

- 1 head dark green lettuce, such as romaine
- 1 bag mixed salad greens
- 7 carrots
- 5 stalks of celery (from the bunch)
- 1 bunch of broccoli
- 1 pint cherry tomatoes or 7 larger tomatoes
- 8 ounces ready-to-eat sunflower seeds

Preparation Before Class

1. Wash the lettuce and the mixed salad greens.

2. Wash the carrots. Keep one carrot whole. If possible, buy a carrot with the top still on and save it for students to observe. Peel and cut the remaining six carrots into thin strips for students to chop.

3. Wash 5 stalks of celery. Keep the rest of the bunch whole for students to observe.

4. Wash and blanch the broccoli. To blanch, place the head of broccoli in boiling water for 1–2 minutes. Rinse and refrigerate immediately. While blanching is not essential, it will make the broccoli a bit softer. This will make it easier to cut with plastic knives. Students may also find it more palatable.

5. Wash the tomatoes. Pick out fruit with stems still attached for students to observe.

6. There is no preparation necessary for the hulled sunflower seeds. Try to bring in a few examples with the seeds still inside the gray "shell."

DIRECTIONS

1. Use your hands to tear the lettuce into bite-sized pieces. Place the lettuce and mixed greens in the salad bowl.

2. With the plastic knife, cut the carrots, celery, broccoli, and tomatoes into bite-sized pieces and place in the salad bowl.

3. Sprinkle a small handful of sunflower seeds over the salad.

4. Gently toss the salad just until it looks mixed. Be careful not to overmix, which may damage the vegetables.

5. Prepare the ***Classroom Salad Dressing*** (see recipe on next page).

6. Serve salad on a plate. Add dressing. Sit, relax, eat, and enjoy.

Composting Scraps: You may wish to save all vegetable scraps and leftover salad for the compost bin you will assemble in Lesson 10. Please rinse any salad that has dressing on it in a colander. These scraps can be saved in the refrigerator or freezer. You can also tear up the paper plates that were used for cutting and add them to the bedding in the compost bin. Do not use plates that have dressing on them in the compost bin. Refer to Lessons 9 and 10 for more information about composting.

Classroom Salad Dressing

Yields 2 cups

INGREDIENTS

2 shallots, minced

2 cloves garlic, minced

3/4 cup olive oil

3/4 cup red wine vinegar

4 tablespoons honey

3 tablespoons Dijon mustard

Salt and pepper

(Optional) 2 sealed containers
or plastic bags

DIRECTIONS

1. Mince the shallots. If you are not using the shallots right away, place them in a sealed container or plastic bag.

2. Mince the garlic. If you are not using the garlic right away, place it in a sealed container or plastic bag.

3. Place the olive oil, vinegar, honey, mustard, minced shallots, and garlic into a bowl. Whisk until thoroughly mixed.

4. Add salt and pepper to taste.

Name   Date

Tomatoes: From Roots to Seeds

When you make a salad, do you ever think about the plant parts that you are eating? Think about it. Lettuce is a leaf. A tomato is a fruit. Carrots are roots. This illustration shows the basic parts of a tomato plant and describes how they help the plant grow. Next time you are in the grocery store, see how many plant parts you can find.

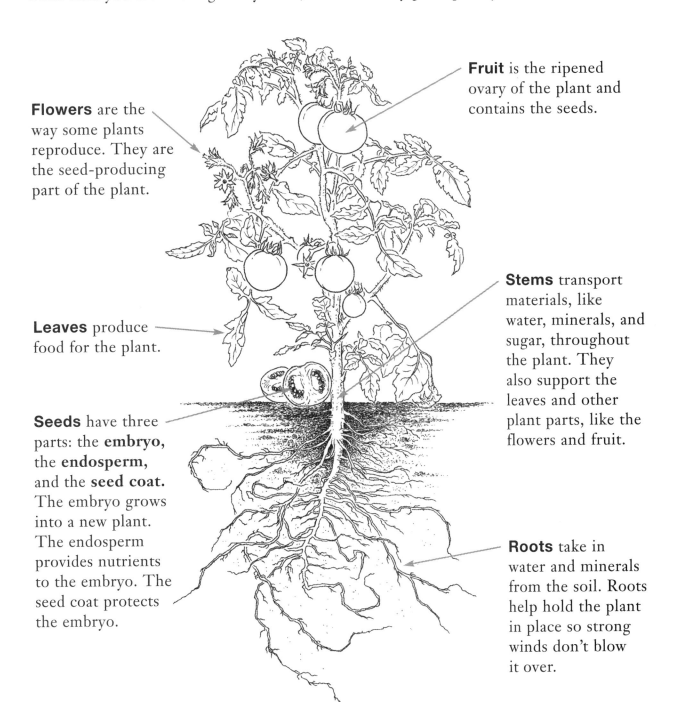

Fruit is the ripened ovary of the plant and contains the seeds.

Flowers are the way some plants reproduce. They are the seed-producing part of the plant.

Leaves produce food for the plant.

Stems transport materials, like water, minerals, and sugar, throughout the plant. They also support the leaves and other plant parts, like the flowers and fruit.

Seeds have three parts: the **embryo**, the **endosperm**, and the **seed coat.** The embryo grows into a new plant. The endosperm provides nutrients to the embryo. The seed coat protects the embryo.

Roots take in water and minerals from the soil. Roots help hold the plant in place so strong winds don't blow it over.

Name   Date

Roots

Structure

There are two major types of root systems. Some plants, like grass, have a fibrous root system. Fibrous roots form a mat-like structure and grow close to the surface of the soil. Other plants, like dandelions, have a taproot system. A taproot system has one main root that reaches deep into the ground. The taproot has a few short side branches.

Function

Roots have two functions for plants. 1) They anchor the plant in place. Think about the roots of a tree or the roots of a carrot plant. The roots of the ivy plant anchor the ivy to a vertical surface, like the side of a building or a wall. 2) They provide moisture and minerals to the plant. Roots that are deep in the ground bring up moisture found there. Surface roots absorb moisture that is closer to the surface. Some roots also store sugar and starches.

Edible Roots

Not all plant roots are edible. Some roots are poisonous. The roots of some vegetable crops are edible, like carrots, beets, and turnips. They are storage roots.

Examples of Edible Roots

Beet
Carrot
Cassava
Horseradish
Lotus root
Parsnip
Rutabaga
Sweet potato
Turnip

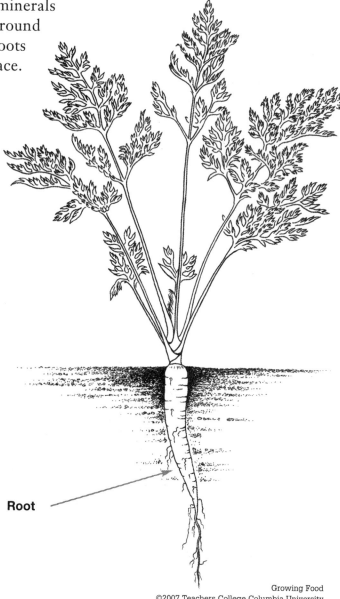

Root

82

LESSON 6: CELEBRATING PLANT PARTS

Growing Food
©2007 Teachers College Columbia University

Name

Date

Stems

Structure

Some stems grow above the ground, like the asparagus in this illustration. Others, like white potatoes, grow below the ground. Stems have structures that act like the veins that move blood in the human vascular system. These tube-like structures in the stem are called **phloem** and **xylem.** They are part of the plant's vascular system.

Function

The stem connects the plant's roots to its leaves. The xylem carries nutrients and water from the roots to other plant parts, including the leaves. The phloem moves the food from the leaves to other parts of the plant. Some stems are modified for storage, like white potatoes. Stems also help support the plant's leaves.

Edible Stems

Look at the list of edible stems. It's hard to believe that some of these are really stems. But they are. For example, white potatoes are a kind of stem called a **tuber.** These are underground stems that store food for the plant.

Examples of Edible Stems

Asparagus
Garlic
Ginger
White potato

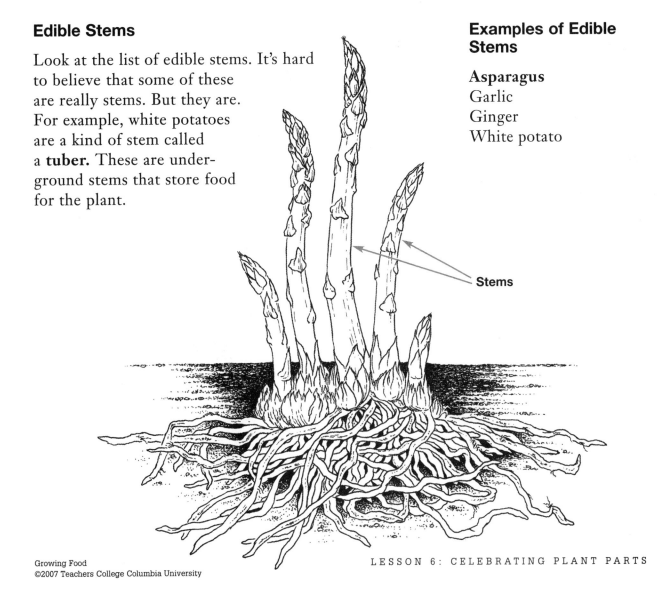

Stems

Growing Food
©2007 Teachers College Columbia University

LESSON 6: CELEBRATING PLANT PARTS

Name	Date

Leaves

Structure

Leaves can be put into two categories: simple and compound. A simple leaf is one blade, or leaf, that connects to the stem by a stalk called the **petiole.** An oak or a maple leaf is a simple leaf. Compound leaves, like clover, are made up of small leaves, or leaflets, that attach to the stem by a petiole. The vascular system found in the stem goes through the petiole and into the leaves. The veins carry water and nutrients from the soil into the leaves and also carry sugars produced by the leaves away from the leaves. The shape of the leaf blade is one way to help identify different kinds of plants.

Function

The main function of leaves is to absorb sunlight to make food through a process called **photosynthesis.** The large flat surface of the leaf makes it possible to absorb lots of light energy from the sun. The plant uses the light energy, carbon dioxide from the air, and water from the soil to make sugars, which are the plant's food.

Edible Leaves

We eat the leaf blade of different kinds of crops. For example, we eat leaves of spinach, parsley, kale, and lettuce. Some of the leaves we eat form a large head, like cabbage, head lettuce, and Brussels sprouts. Some of the bulbs we eat, like leeks and onions, are really clusters of leaves. The celery stalk we eat is the petiole that joins the celery leaves to the stem.

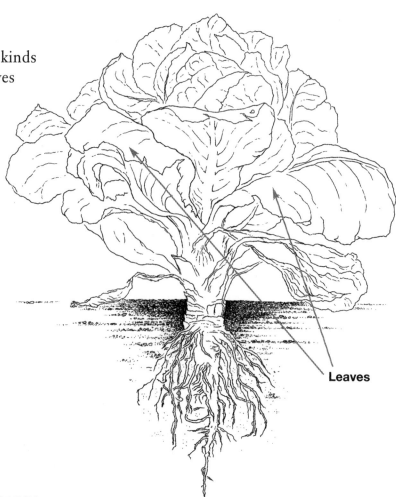

Leaves

Examples of Edible Leaves

Cabbage	Mustard
Collards	Parsley
Kale	Spinach
Lettuce	

LESSON 6: CELEBRATING PLANT PARTS

Name   Date

Flowers

Structure

The parts of a flower are the **pistil**, the **stamen**, the **sepals**, and the **petals**. The pistil is the female reproductive part. It is usually found in the center of the flower. It has three parts: the **stigma**, the **style**, and the **ovary**. The stigma is at the top of the pistil. It is attached to the style, a long, tube-like structure. The style leads to the ovary, which contains the female egg cells, called **ovules**. After the egg is fertilized, the ovule develops into a seed. The stamen is the male reproductive part of the flower. It is made up of the **anther**, a pollen sac, and a long filament. The filament holds the anther in place so the pollen can be scattered by the wind or carried away by **pollinators**, like insects, bats, or birds. The sepals are green leaf-like structures at the base of the flower that protect the bud. The **petals** are the colorful part of the flower and are often fragrant.

Function

Even though flowers may be pretty to look at, their primary function is for reproduction. Seeds are formed when pollen moves from an anther to a stigma. The fragrant petals attract pollinators that help transfer the pollen. The pollen lands on the stigma and moves down the tube-like style and enters the ovary. If pollination is successful, the male sperm cells fertilize the ovules, which develop into seeds. The ovary becomes the fruit.

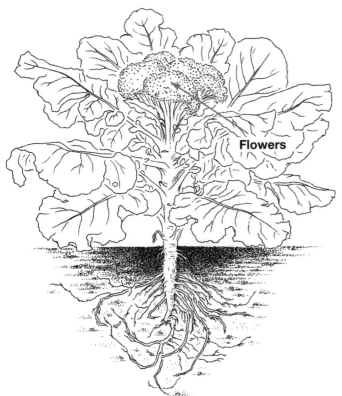

Flowers

Edible Flowers

Not all flowers are edible. It's important to know which ones are and to check before you eat any flowers. Only eat flowers that are grown as a crop. Eating flowers was very popular during Victorian times and has even been traced back to Roman times. Some edible flowers are used to make flavored vinegars. Some flowers, like squash blossoms, are perfect for stuffing.

Examples of Edible Flowers

Borage	Garlic blossoms
Broccoli	Nasturtiums
Calendula	Squash blossoms
Chive blossoms	Violets

Name   Date

Fruit

Structure

The scientific meaning of the word "fruit" is not the same as the everyday one. When most people think of fruit, they think of a food, like apples, bananas, or strawberries. When scientists talk about fruit, they mean the part of the plant that surrounds one or more seeds. Fruit like apples and tomatoes have flesh that surrounds the seeds. However, some kinds of fruit, like Brazil nuts, do not have soft flesh. The nut's hard shell is the fruit, and the seed inside is what we eat.

Function

Fruits help in spreading seeds. For example, colorful, fragrant fruit is attractive to animals. The animals eat the ripe flesh, including the seeds. The seeds survive the digestion process and end up in the animal droppings on top of soil. A new plant begins to grow, and the life cycle starts all over again.

Edible Fruit

Not all fruits are edible. We don't eat the dry pods of milkweed or the winged fruits of the maple. But there are many kinds of fruit that we do eat. These include berries, avocados, cucumbers, olives, and many more. Some of the spices we use, like nutmeg and allspice, are also fruits.

Examples of Edible Fruit

Apples   Peppers
Cucumbers   Pumpkins
Grapes   String beans
Peaches   **Tomatoes**
Pears

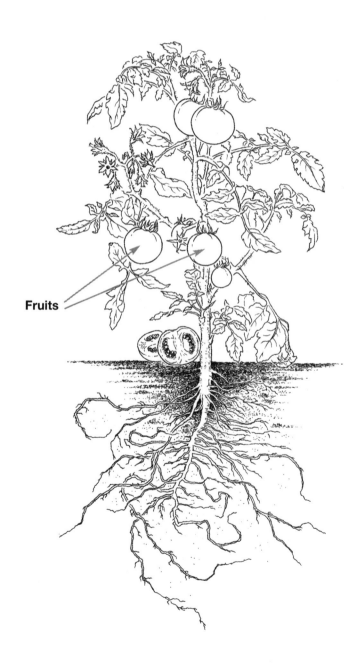

Fruits

LESSON 6: CELEBRATING PLANT PARTS   Growing Food
©2007 Teachers College Columbia University

BECOMING FOOD SCIENTISTS : PLANTS : FOOD WEBS : AGRICULTURE : MAKING CHOICES

Name   Date

Seeds

Structure

A seed contains all that is needed for a new plant to grow. Seeds have three basic parts: the **embryo,** the **endosperm,** and the **seed coat.** The embryo inside the seed develops into the new plant. The endosperm is the stored food that nourishes the embryo when it begins to develop. The seed coat protects the embryo until conditions such as temperature and moisture are right for the plant to begin to grow.

Function

Seeds are the way plants can increase their populations. A major function of the seed is to protect the embryo until conditions are right for the plant to begin to grow. Since plants cannot move to new locations to live and grow, they have to have ways of scattering their seeds to new places where they can grow. There are lots of different ways that seeds "travel." How they travel depends on the properties of the seeds. Some seeds travel on the wind, others float in the water, and still others "hitchhike" by sticking to animal fur or human clothing. Sometimes animals like squirrels carry the seeds to new locations and bury them. When the time is right, the new plants begin to grow.

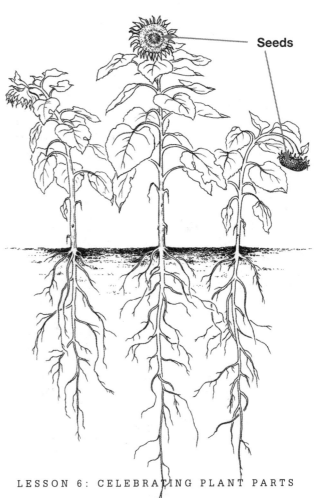

Seeds

Edible Seeds

Seeds also include the food we call "nuts." When you eat almonds, Brazil nuts, cashews, or macadamias, you crack open the hard fruit to get to the kernel, or seed. Sunflower seeds are the seeds you find inside the grayish "husk." Not all seeds are edible. Some are poisonous and some may have been treated with chemicals. Never eat seeds from a garden seed packet. Be sure to check with an adult before you eat any seeds.

Examples of Edible Seeds

Almonds	Peas
Brazil nuts	Pumpkin seeds
Cashews	**Sunflower seeds**

BECOMING FOOD SCIENTISTS : PLANTS : FOOD WEBS : AGRICULTURE : MAKING CHOICES

Name		Date

Plant Parts We Eat

List as many edible roots, stems, leaves, flowers, fruit, and seeds as you can. You can ask your family and friends for help.

Plant Parts We Eat		
Roots	**Stems**	**Leaves**
Flowers	**Fruit**	**Seeds**

LESSON 6: CELEBRATING PLANT PARTS

Name	Date

Take-Home Salad

Serves 4–6

In class we have been learning about plants and plant parts. To celebrate what we have learned, we made a plant-part salad using a recipe like this one. Take this recipe home and make it with your family. Share what you learned about plant parts with your family.

SALAD INGREDIENTS

1 head of a dark green lettuce such as romaine or 1 bag mixed salad greens

2 carrots, cut into thin slices by an adult

2 stalks celery

1/2 bunch of broccoli

2 tomatoes

2 ounces ready-to-eat sunflower seeds

DRESSING INGREDIENTS (OPTIONAL)

Yield 2 cups

3/4 cup olive oil

3/4 cup red wine vinegar

4 tablespoons honey

3 tablespoons Dijon mustard

2 shallots, minced

2 cloves garlic, minced

Salt and pepper to taste

MATERIALS

1 large salad bowl

1 sturdy plastic knife

1 cutting board

1 vegetable peeler

1 colander

DIRECTIONS

1. Thoroughly wash all vegetables to remove any soil that may still be on them from the farm.

2. Use your hands to tear the lettuce into bite-sized pieces. Place the lettuce in the salad bowl.

3. Use a vegetable peeler to peel the carrots.

4. Use a plastic knife to cut the carrots, celery, broccoli, and tomatoes into bite-sized pieces. Place them in the salad bowl.

5. Take a small handful of sunflower seeds and gently sprinkle them over the salad.

6. Carefully toss the salad just until it looks mixed. Be careful not to overmix. You don't want to damage the vegetables.

7. (Optional) If you are making dressing, place all ingredients in a bowl and mix with a whisk.

8. Serve the salad on a plate. Add salad dressing as desired, saving leftover dressing for future salads.

9. Sit, relax, eat, and enjoy.

Energy Transformation

AIM

To gain an understanding of photosynthesis and how plants provide animals with food.

SCIENTIFIC PROCESSES

question, investigate, search, construct knowledge

OBJECTIVES

Students will be able to:

- discuss the process of photosynthesis;

- describe how food energy produced in the leaves travels to seeds;

- value plants for their ability to capture and store energy from the sun.

OVERVIEW

In this lesson students continue their exploration of the Unit 2 Question. Through an investigation and a series of readings, students are introduced to energy and matter transformations in the process of photosynthesis. These are complex topics for adults as well as for students. To help make this information accessible, we chose a popular food, peanuts, as the thread that weaves the concepts together. Most students have eaten peanuts or peanut butter. In fact, you may find that they already think of peanuts as a high-energy snack. However, they may not realize that the energy we get from eating peanuts is stored energy the peanut plant gets from the sun. Students may need to be reminded that energy can change form. In photosynthesis, light energy from the sun is transformed to stored chemical energy that can be used by living organisms, like the peanut plant and its seeds (the peanuts). We begin with a reading about energy and close with a detailed look at photosynthesis.

Alert: Before you begin this lesson, make sure no one is allergic to peanuts. See the *Energy Burn* experiment sheet for other options.

MATERIALS

For the teacher:
- *Energy Transformation* sample conversation
- *Energy Burn* experiment sheet
- *Photosynthesis Review Answer Sheet* lesson resource
- *Food for Thought* teacher note
- *Six Steps to an Experiment* lesson resource (p. 38)
- Overhead transparency film
- Transparency markers
- Overhead projector
- Chart paper
- Markers

For the class:
- 5 dry-roasted peanuts
- 1 potato
- Paper clip

- Matches

For each student:
- *What's Energy?* student reading
- *A Brief History of Peanuts* student reading
- *How Peanuts Grow* student reading
- *The Peanut Plant* student reading
- *Roots Close Up* student reading
- *Stem Close Up* student reading
- *Leaves Close Up* student reading
- *How Plants Make Food* student reading
- *Inside a Leaf* student reading
- *Photosynthesis Review* activity sheet
- LiFE Logs

PROCEDURE

Before You Begin:

- Review the *Energy Transformation* sample conversation.

- Review the *Energy Burn* experiment sheet and gather together the materials.

- Make an overhead transparency of the peanut-plant drawing found on the *Peanut Plant* student reading.

- Make copies of the student readings.

- If you have not already done so, post the Module Question and the Unit 2 Question at the front of the class.

MODULE QUESTION

How does nature provide us with food?

UNIT QUESTION

If there were no plants, would humans have food?

 SEARCHING

1. Read about Energy and Peanuts

Engage students in a brief discussion of energy to check for student understanding. *What's energy? Can you name some different kinds of energy?* (Sound, light, heat, chemical, mechanical.) *Where does energy come from?* Accept all answers. Record them on the chart paper. If food did not come up in your energy discussion, introduce food as a source of energy. *How many of you eat peanuts as a snack? Peanut-butter sandwiches? Why do you eat these?* If no one includes energy in his or her response, introduce the idea of getting energy from food. *Let's do some research to learn more about energy and peanuts.*

Method 1: Distribute *What's Energy?, How Peanuts Grow*, and *A Brief History of Peanuts* to students. After students complete *What's*

Energy?, refer back to the chart paper. *Does anyone want to change anything on this list? Are there new ideas that you would like to add?* Keep the list and refer to it through this lesson.

Next, have students read *A Brief History of Peanuts.* You may wish to have students take turns reading paragraphs out loud. Finally, read *How Peanuts Grow.* Check for student understanding of the word "food." The everyday meaning of food is something "taken in." But the scientific meaning of food is substances from which living organisms get energy to carry out their life processes, and the materials, or building blocks, from which they are made. Given this scientific meaning of food, check for student understanding that plants make their food rather than taking it in. Given that plants take in water and nutrients from the soil, people often consider these materials "plant food."

With each drawing of the peanut plant, ask students to describe how the plant gets food. *Does a seed need food? Where does the food come from? Where is the plant getting food?* Accept all answers. If students have different ideas, point out that in this lesson the class will be investigating questions about plants and how they get food. Invite students to share new information they have learned about peanuts. Add this to the chart paper.

Method 2: Divide the class into three groups: Food Scientists, Food Historians, and Botanists. Each group will read one of the student readings and report back to the class. For example, the Food Scientists will read *What's Energy?,* the Food Historians will read *A Brief History of Peanuts,* and the Botanists will read *How Peanuts Grow.* Guide the student readings as described in Method 1. If you choose this method, assign all three readings as homework.

2. Review the Module and Unit Questions

Remind students of the Unit Question. Explain that in this lesson the class is going to continue its explorations of the question and how plants get food. To begin the explorations, students are going to do an investigation. The investigation was designed to try to answer the question, *Do peanuts have energy?*

3. LiFE Logs

Have students take out their LiFE Logs and write, "Do peanuts have energy?" Next, have students write their predictions. Remind students to describe what they are basing their predictions on. Note: Students have just read *What's Energy?* and discussed that the energy stored in peanuts is released inside our bodies when we eat them. The investigation that students will perform in *Energy Burn* provides evidence to support the fact that peanuts have stored energy.

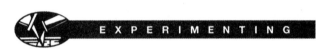

4. Conduct Energy Burn Investigation

As you set up the investigation using the *Energy Burn* experiment sheet, review *Six Steps to an Experiment*. *What is the question we want to answer? What do we predict?* Review the materials and methods with students. Ask students to record what they observe in their LiFE Logs.

 THEORIZING

5. Discuss Observations

Use the questions on the experiment sheet to guide this discussion. If necessary, burn another peanut and conduct a guided discussion. As the peanut is burning, remind students that they are seeing the stored energy in the peanut, which is a seed, being released as heat and light. Help students understand that burning the peanut is one way to demonstrate that the peanut has stored energy and that energy is transformed from chemical energy to light and heat energy. Ask, *What would happen to the energy in the peanut if we did not burn it?* (If we planted

a raw peanut, it would grow into a plant. If we ate the peanut, we would get the energy from the peanut.)

6. Construct Knowledge about Photosynthesis

Distribute *The Peanut Plant, Roots Close Up, Stem Close Up, Leaves Close Up, How Plants Make Food,* and *Inside a Leaf* student readings. Give students a few minutes to look over the materials. Explain that now the class is going to learn more about how peanut plants and peanut seeds — the part of the plant we eat — get energy and where the energy we observed when we burned the peanut came from. Invite students to take turns reading and discussing the material out loud. Through a guided discussion, help students understand the process of photosynthesis.

Challenge students to think about how plants get food. Encourage them to think about what they have already learned about plants and structure and function. Direct their reading through questioning them about the peanut-plant parts. *What do the roots do? Where is the stem? What does the stem do? What do the peanut plant leaves look like? What happens in the leaves? How do you know?* Connect this to the *Blocking the Light* and *Blocking the Stomata* experiments. *What evidence do we have from our own classroom experiments that supports the idea that plants make their own food?* Make it clear that all ideas and thoughts are welcome. The sample conversation and teacher note can help you guide your students through this discussion.

Distribute the *Photosynthesis Review* activity sheet. After students have completed the answers, discuss as a class.

7. LiFE Logs

Ask students to describe the process of photosynthesis in their own words.

Energy Transformation

This sample conversation in the **Theorizing** phase of the QuESTA cycle will help you guide your students through a conversation that will enable them to construct new knowledge. As you engage students in your own conversation, encourage them to debate the interpretation of the results of their experiment, to explain their own theories about what they learned, and to recognize how they might use this new knowledge in their daily lives. This is a guide. Feel free to adjust your questioning to the needs of your class.

MS. D: When we burned the peanut we learned that a peanut has energy in it. In the last lesson, we discussed the fact that plants use energy from the sun to make food. *When you look at this drawing of a peanut plant leaf, can you tell me how the energy from the sun might get into the plant?*

BEN: I see an arrow that shows light going to the leaf of the plant.

MS. D: Yes, light energy from the sun enters plants through the leaves. Look at the picture of the leaf again. *Does anyone see anything else that goes into the leaf?*

LINDA: I see an arrow that shows carbon dioxide from the air going into the leaf and I see another arrow from the stem that shows water going into the leaf.

MS. D: So, in the leaf we have light energy, carbon dioxide from the air, and water. Look at the picture. *What does the leaf make with these?*

BEN: On the drawing it says the leaf makes sugar.

MS. D: Yes, as Ben said, the plant makes sugar using light energy from the sun, water from the soil, and carbon dioxide from the air. This process is called photosynthesis. *Can someone explain photosynthesis using your own words?*

LINDA: The leaf of the plant turns toward the sun and gets energy. The leaf also gets carbon dioxide from the air and water that came in through the stem. The energy, carbon dioxide, and water turn into sugar. The light energy the plant got from the sun is inside the sugar.

MS. D: Very good. The sugar has the sun's energy in it. *Now, how does the energy get to the peanut?*

LINDA: Maybe the sugar travels through the stem from the leaf to the peanut, just like the water travels from the root up to the leaves.

MS. D: Yes, the sugar made in the leaves travels throughout the plant to help it grow. Since the peanut is a seed, the plant stores enough energy there so the seed can grow into a plant.

BEN: Hey, I got it! The heat and light from the sun go into the plant, and then when we burned the peanut, we saw the heat and the light come back out again.

MS. D: Yes, we saw the energy come out of the peanut as light and heat energy. Remember, when the energy was in the peanut it was stored as chemical energy.

Energy Burn

Warning: Before you bring peanuts into your classroom, make sure no one is allergic to them. If you have a student with a peanut allergy, try burning a tree nut (Brazil nut, cashew, almond) or a cracker.

This experiment will help students understand that peanuts, a plant-based food, contain energy. Plants make their food through the process of photosynthesis. Plants use energy from the sun to change carbon dioxide and water into sugars. The sugars provide the energy and the building blocks that plants need to live and grow. When the peanut burns, it releases the stored energy as heat energy and light energy.

Setup

1. Place the paper clip on a flat surface.

2. Bend the top half of the paper clip up and straighten the lower half, as shown in the drawing.

3. Make the bottom half of the paper clip as straight as possible.

4. Place one peanut in the "cradle" formed by the bent paper clip.

5. Push the straight edge of the paper clip into the potato.

Procedure

1. Make sure the peanut is secure in the "cradle."

2. Light the match. It may take 2–4 matches to ignite the peanut. Once it is ignited, the peanut will burn for 2–3 minutes.

3. Watch the peanut carefully through the entire burning. If it looks as if it might fall off the cradle, blow it out.

Questions

1. *When something burns, what is released? Think about what you feel when you stand close to a fire.*

2. Watch the peanut burn. *What do you see?*

3. *Where do the light and the heat come from?*

4. *Where did the peanut get the light and the heat?*

5. *If we didn't burn the peanut, what would happen to the stored energy?*

6. (When the fire goes out) *What made the fire go out?*

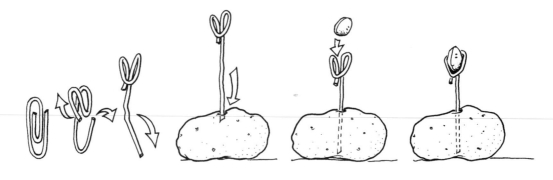

Photosynthesis Review Answer Sheet

1. Plants use *[ENERGY]* from the *[SUN]*, *[CARBON DIOXIDE]* from the *[AIR]*, and *[WATER]* from the *[SOIL]* in the process called photosynthesis.

2. Plants make their own *[FOOD]* through photosynthesis.

3. The scientific meaning of the word "food" is: a source of *[ENERGY]* and *[BUILDING BLOCKS]* that organisms need to live and grow.

4. During photosynthesis, *[LIGHT]* energy from the sun is changed into *[CHEMICAL]* energy that is stored inside sugar.

5. During photosynthesis, carbon dioxide and water are changed to *[SUGAR]*; *[OXYGEN]* is given off as waste.

6. Photosynthesis takes place inside the cells that have *[CHLOROPLASTS]*.

7. *[CHLOROPHYLL]* is a green pigment that gives plants their green color.

8. When animals, including humans, eat plants, they are using the food the plants made. This gives their body a source of *[ENERGY]* and the *[BUILDING BLOCKS]* they need to live and grow.

Food for Thought

Think about the number of times you've read in a textbook that one of the differences between plants and animals is that plants make their own food. It seems clear enough. Animals take food into their bodies by eating. Plants make their own food using a process called photosynthesis. There may even be a brief description of photosynthesis in those textbooks. How plants make food, the release of energy from food, and the flow of energy and matter through a food web are all common topics in middle school science texts. Your students may even be familiar with all the terminology. The question is, do they really understand it?

Research on student learning indicates that they may not. In evaluating curriculum materials, Project 2061, the AAAS's long-term initiative to improve literacy in science, math, and technology, has found that many materials are not successful in helping students understand important concepts. In part, some of the difficulties students have are due to the words "food" and "energy." The definition of "energy" is the ability to do work. The definition of "food" is a bit more complicated. The everyday meaning of "food" is something we take into our body. The scientific meaning is a source of fuel and a source of structural materials or building blocks.

In addition to students' naive views, on the Web site of the American Institute of Biological Sciences, David R. Hershey, a biology education consultant, reports that the teaching literature contains hundreds of errors or misconceptions about plants, including the explanation of photosynthesis. Many of the misconceptions are due to oversimplifying the explanations. How to help upper elementary and middle school students understand photosynthesis is challenging. While you don't want to oversimplify, you also don't want to provide complex definitions or formulas that students memorize but don't comprehend. Let your students' prior knowledge of science guide the level of complexity you introduce. Keep the information accurate and age-appropriate.

Consider using reflective writing to uncover students' thinking about plants, food, photosynthesis, and energy transformation. Ask students to respond to the question: *What are the raw materials plants use to make food?* Have students record their thinking in their LiFE Logs at the beginning of the lesson and again at the end. Did their thinking change? Thinking about the process of photosynthesis will help shift the focus away from an exercise of naming products or memorizing labels.

When you think about it, green plants really are rather remarkable. What else produces the oxygen that animals, including people, need to breathe? What else can transform light energy into chemical energy stored in food? What else produces the energy and matter all living things need to grow and survive? Without green plants, where would we be?

Name   Date

What's Energy?

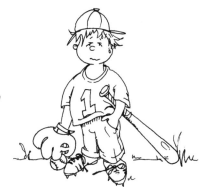

We use the word **energy** all the time. We talk about running out of energy. *I don't have enough energy to do any more.* We talk about saving energy. *Turn off that light to save energy.* Sometimes we talk about the energy in food. *Eat more pasta because it's full of energy.* But what exactly is energy?

Just about everything has energy in it. Plants have energy. The sun has energy. Our bodies have energy from the food we eat. Even a tiny peanut has energy stored inside it. We call this **chemical energy.**

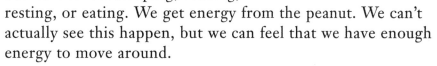

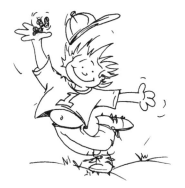

When we eat a peanut, the stored energy inside the peanut is released inside our bodies so we can do **work.** Sometimes that work is running, jumping, and playing. Sometimes it is sleeping, reading, resting, or eating. We get energy from the peanut. We can't actually see this happen, but we can feel that we have enough energy to move around.

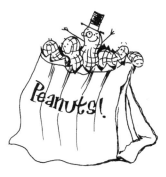

If we can't see it happen, how do we know that peanuts really have energy? We can set up an experiment to try to answer our question: *Do peanuts have energy?* Before we do our experiment, think about how we can tell when energy is being released in our bodies. What happens when you run, jump, and play for a long time?

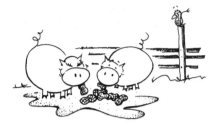

Name   Date

A Brief History of Peanuts

What do goobers, guinea seeds, ground peas, ground nuts, and monkey nuts all have in common? They are all different names for the same food — peanuts!

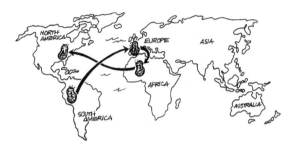

The peanut plant has been around for a long, long time. Archaeologists have found evidence that peanut plants were growing in Brazil, and possibly other parts of South America, more than 3,000 years ago. European explorers brought the peanut plant from South America back to Europe. Traders took peanut plants to parts of Asia and Africa. Eventually, peanut plants were brought from Africa to North America and planted in the southern United States. Peanut plants now grow in warm regions around the world.

Until the Civil War, peanuts were a food associated with the southern United States. However, during the Civil War, both Union and Confederate soldiers used the peanut as food during hard times.

In 1870 P. T. Barnum introduced hot roasted peanuts as a snack food at his show, which later became the Barnum and Bailey Circus. They were a hit. Everyone loved them. As the circus traveled from town to town, the peanut became more popular. Soon roasted peanuts began showing up at baseball games and theaters. In fact, the cheap seats in theaters were called the "peanut galleries."

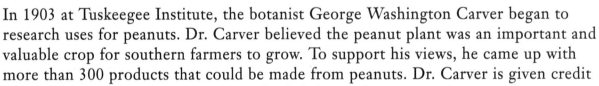

In 1903 at Tuskeegee Institute, the botanist George Washington Carver began to research uses for peanuts. Dr. Carver believed the peanut plant was an important and valuable crop for southern farmers to grow. To support his views, he came up with more than 300 products that could be made from peanuts. Dr. Carver is given credit

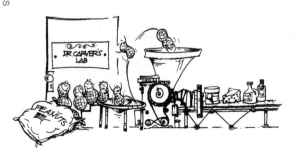

for helping make peanuts the second most important crop grown in the South. Today, some of the most popular products in the United States are peanuts, peanut butter, and peanut candy. The American Peanut Council reports that the average American eats more than 6 pounds of peanuts and peanut products each year.

BECOMING FOOD SCIENTISTS : **PLANTS** : FOOD WEBS : AGRICULTURE : MAKING CHOICES

Name   Date

How Peanuts Grow

Did you know that peanuts are not really nuts? They are **legumes,** and they belong to the same plant family, *Leguminosae,* as beans and peas. Legumes are edible seeds inside a pod.

Peanut plants grow from kernels, or seeds. In the United States, most of the peanuts we eat are grown in New Mexico, Texas, Oklahoma, Alabama, Florida, Georgia, South Carolina, North Carolina, and Virginia. The kernels usually are planted several weeks after the last frost, most often between April and the first week of June. After a few days the young seedlings send out roots and the first leaves begin to grow. For the first few weeks, the roots, stems, and leaves continue to grow. About one month after planting the seeds, the first flowers appear.

The peanut plant flowers don't need pollinators because they pollinate themselves, or **self-pollinate.** The petals fall off the flowers and the fertilized ovary begins to grow larger. The ovary forms a small stem called a **peg.** The peanut embryo is in the tip of the peg, which grows downward into the soil. The soil has to be moist enough for the peg to be able to push into it.

Underground, the peanut embryo begins to take the shape of a peanut pod. Inside the pods, the seeds begin to grow. There usually are two to five seeds per pod. It takes two to three months from the time the peanut kernels are planted for seeds to begin to grow. The seeds continue to grow until they fill the inside of the pod. We eat these seeds, which we call peanuts. Peanuts need about four months to grow before they are ready to harvest.

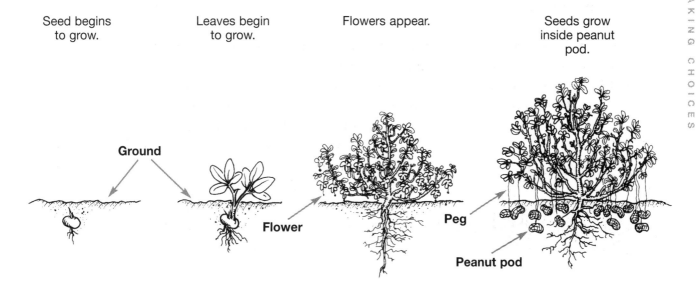

Seed begins to grow.   Leaves begin to grow.   Flowers appear.   Seeds grow inside peanut pod.

Ground

Flower

Peg

Peanut pod

Name   Date

The Peanut Plant

Arachis hypogea

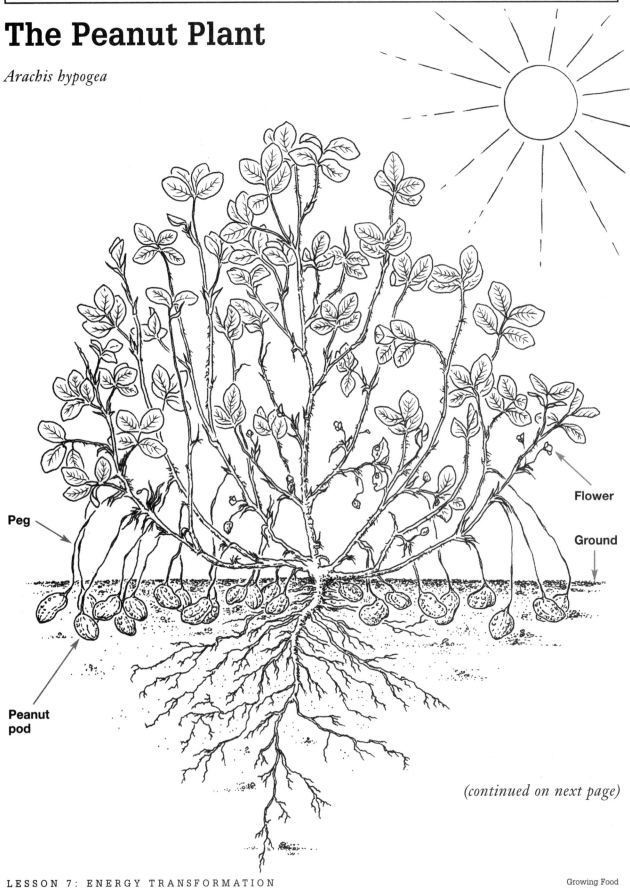

Peg

Flower

Ground

Peanut
pod

(continued on next page)

Growing Food
©2007 Teachers College Columbia University

BECOMING FOOD SCIENTISTS : **PLANTS** : FOOD WEBS : AGRICULTURE : MAKING CHOICES

Name   Date

The Peanut Plant

Look closely at the illustration of the peanut plant. Like most plants, it lives in two different environments. Its roots live in the soil, and its stems and leaves live above the ground. Green plants grow in light. They take in light energy and transform it into the chemical energy found in sugars. This process is called **photosynthesis.** During photosynthesis, carbon dioxide and water are changed to sugars and oxygen. The sugars are food and travel throughout the plant to reach all the plant's cells. The plant gives off the oxygen as waste. The energy-containing food that is not used is stored to be used at some other time. Different plants store this extra energy in different places. For example, the peanut plant stores some of its excess energy in the seeds, or "peanuts," it produces. When you eat the peanuts, you are eating some of the plant's stored energy.

Plants are unique. They are not like animals. Plants are **producers.** They make their own food, and what they don't use, they store. Think about the scientific meaning of the word "food." When scientists talk about food, they mean the energy that a living organism needs to carry out its life processes and the material, or building blocks, that the living organism is made of. This means that the plant's food, the sugars the plant makes, is what gives the plant both the energy and the building blocks it needs to live and grow.

Think about the ways that animals, including humans, benefit from photosynthesis. For example, grass makes its own food. Then cows eat the grass and produce milk. The cows use some of the food energy from the grass to grow and reproduce. Some of the energy is given off as heat. And some of the food energy is stored in their milk. We milk the cows and make dairy products that we can eat or drink, like butter, cheese, and milk. We get food energy from the dairy products. Can you think of other ways that animals benefit from photosynthesis? Think about an insect that eats a plant, like grass. What if a frog eats that insect and a snake eats that frog and a hawk eats that snake? Do you think the plant — grass — benefits all the animals? Think about what might happen if there were no plants. Now think about the Module Question, *How does nature provide us with food?*

DID YOU KNOW...?

Photo means "light"
Synthesis means "put together"

Name   Date

Roots Close Up

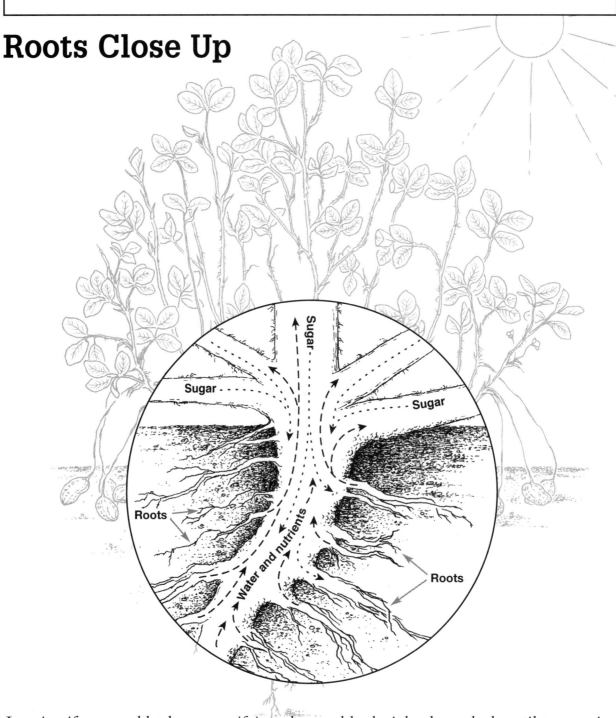

Imagine if you could take a magnifying glass and look right through the soil to examine a peanut plant growing underground. You would see the large taproot with many smaller roots growing off to the sides. Notice how many roots there are and how they are growing. These roots absorb water and nutrients from the soil. They also hold the plant firmly in the ground. Roots also have another function — to store energy. Some roots are edible, like turnips and carrots. Edible roots are a source of food for other living things, like rabbits, pigs, and humans.

Name   Date

Stem Close Up

Now take your magnifying glass and use it to examine the peanut plant's stem. The stem connects the roots and the leaves. Notice how it supports the plant leaves in the air. The stem carries water and nutrients from the roots to other parts of the plant, including the leaves. The stem has two structures that help carry the water and the energy-containing food throughout the plant. One structure transports the food — sugar — from the leaves to other parts of the plant. Sometimes the sugars flow upward to the flower or fruit, and sometimes they flow downward toward the roots. The other structure transports the water and nutrients from the roots through the plant. Some kinds of stems, like white potatoes, store excess food energy from the plant.

Name   Date

Leaves Close Up

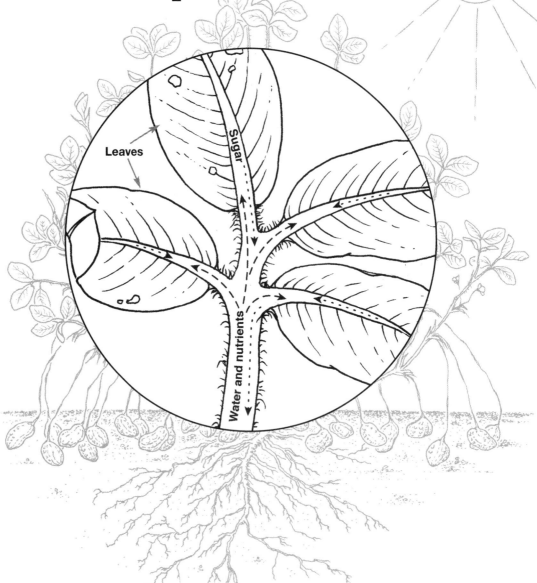

If you could take your magnifying glass and look at the peanut plant's leaves, you would see groups of four oval-shaped leaves attached to the stem. The main function of a plant's leaves is to produce energy-containing food through photosynthesis. The shape and structure of a leaf are adaptations that make photosynthesis possible. Leaves have veins that carry the water and nutrients from the stem to the leaves, and sugar from the leaves to the rest of the plant.

Not all plants have leaves for photosynthesis. For example, the leaves on cacti are called **spines.** They are sharp and protect the plant. Photosynthesis takes place in the cactus stem instead of the leaves.

LESSON 7: ENERGY TRANSFORMATION

Growing Food
©2007 Teachers College Columbia University

How Plants Make Food

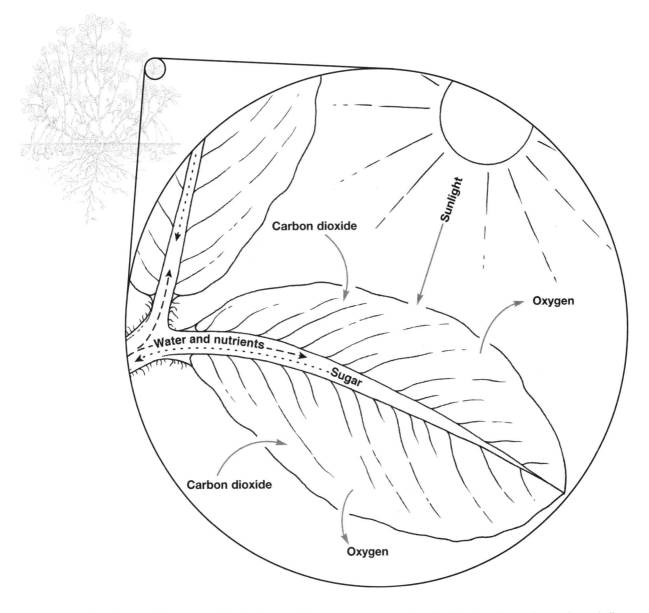

Look closely at this magnified view of a peanut plant leaf. Notice how broad and flat it is. Because of this shape, a large area is exposed to the sun. Green plants make their own food through a process called photosynthesis. Plants absorb light energy from the sun, take in carbon dioxide from the air through their leaves, and water and nutrients from the soil through their roots. The plant uses the light energy, carbon dioxide, water, and nutrients to make sugars that are the plant's food. Some of the food energy is used by the plant, some is released as heat, and some food energy is stored. Other organisms that eat the plant use this stored energy. During the process of photosynthesis, the plant gives off oxygen, which is released into the air.

Name   Date

Inside a Leaf

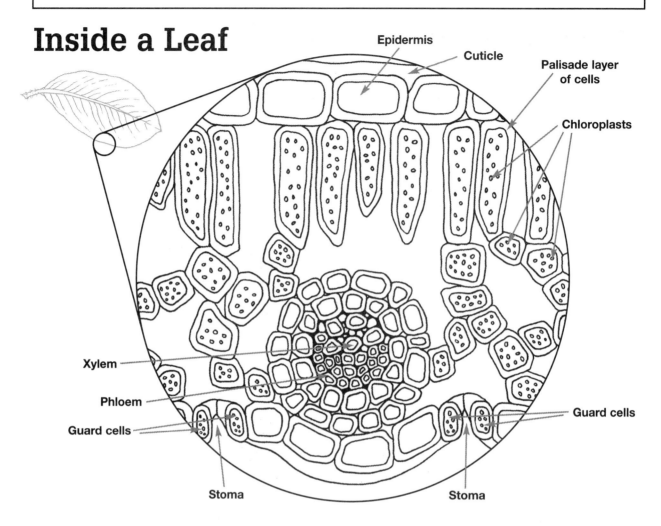

Think about how thin most leaves are. Now, imagine you are looking at a peanut plant leaf with a very powerful microscope. You would be observing the leaf's cellular structure. This is a drawing of what you might see. Find the **epidermis.** It is the leaf's protective, outer layer of cells. The **cuticle,** a waxy, transparent layer that acts as a waterproof covering, covers the epidermis. The epidermis and the cuticle keep water and gases from moving through the leaf. So how does carbon dioxide get in and oxygen and water move out? Find the **stomata** (plural of **stoma**). These are the narrow openings in the leaf that let gases move into the leaf and oxygen and water move out. The stomata have **guard cells** that control the opening and closing of the stomata.

Look for the **chloroplasts.** Inside the chloroplasts is the pigment **chlorophyll,** which gives plants their green color. Photosynthesis takes place in the cells that have chloroplasts. You'll see that most of the chloroplasts are in the **palisade layer** of cells just below the leaf's top surface. Can you guess why? You guessed it — since the sun is overhead, most of the light hits the top surface. Inside the vein, there is the **xylem,** which carries water and minerals, and the **phloem,** which carries the food.

LESSON 7: ENERGY TRANSFORMATION

Name	Date

Photosynthesis Review

1. Plants use _____ from the _____,

_____ from the _____, and

_____ from the _____ in the process called

photosynthesis.

2. Plants make their own _____ through photosynthesis.

3. The scientific meaning of the word "food" is: a source of _____

and _____ that organisms need to live and grow.

4. During photosynthesis, _____ energy from the sun is changed

into _____ energy that is stored inside sugar.

5. During photosynthesis, carbon dioxide and water are changed to

_____. _____ is given off as waste.

6. Photosynthesis takes place inside the cells that have _____.

7. _____ is a green pigment that gives plants their green color.

8. When animals, including humans, eat plants, they are using the food the plants

made. This gives their body a source of _____ and the

_____ they need to live and grow.

Linking Plants and Animals

AIM

To understand how feeding relationships link plants and animals.

SCIENTIFIC PROCESSES

- **construct knowledge, build theories**

OBJECTIVES

Students will be able to:

- **respond to the Unit 2 Question and cite evidence to support their answer;**

- **discuss why all animals, including humans, depend on plants for food;**

- **explain the terms "producers" and "consumers";**

- **demonstrate understanding of the interdependent nature of living things.**

OVERVIEW

Throughout this unit students have been learning about plants and how they make their own food. In this culminating lesson, students synthesize what they have learned thus far about plants as producers and are introduced to the role of consumers. Students also consider how feeding relationships link plants and animals in a biological community. Students learn that food chains are a way to represent the flow of energy and matter from one organism to another. They learn that food chains only show one possible source of food for an animal. As a class activity, students make a bulletin-board display that models a simple food chain. The lesson concludes with students reflecting on what they have learned and answering the Unit 2 Question in their LiFE Logs. In Unit 3, students will continue their investigations of feeding relationships and discover how food chains are linked together to make more complex food webs.

MATERIALS

For the teacher:
- *Who Eats What Food?* lesson resource
- *Understanding Food Chains* teacher note

For the class:
- Chart paper
- *The Peanut Plant* student reading (pp. 100–101)
- 5 skeins of different-colored yarn

- Scissors
- Pushpins
- 5 index cards
- 5 red or orange markers
- 5 blue or black markers

For each student:
- LiFE Log

PROCEDURE

Before You Begin:

- Review *Who Eats What Food?* lesson resource for more suggestions of organisms to include in the food chain activity.

- On chart paper, write the names of the members of the food chain from *The Peanut Plant* student reading in Lesson 7: grass, insect, frog, snake, hawk.

- Review *Understanding Food Chains* teacher note.

- If you have not already done so, post the Module Question and the Unit 2 Question at the front of the class.

MODULE QUESTION

How does nature provide us with food?

UNIT QUESTION

If there were no plants, would humans have food?

 THEORIZING

1. Review the Module and Unit Questions

Tell students that this is the final lesson in Unit 2. In this lesson, they will think through what they have learned and discuss their ideas about answers to the Module and Unit questions.

2. Reconsider Food Chains

Review the description of the food chain from *The Peanut Plant* student reading in Lesson 7. Post the chart paper with the names of the members of this food chain recorded on it. Explain to students that there are three major categories of living organisms in an ecosystem. In this lesson, they will focus on two of them: producers and consumers. *What's the definition of a producer? What's the definition of a consumer?*

3. Discuss Consumers

Return to the list of organisms on the chart paper. *Are there any producers on this list? Do you see any consumers on the list?* Write "producer" or "consumer" next to each organism. Write "consumers" at the top of a separate sheet of chart paper and make three columns. Invite students to brainstorm a list of consumers and some of the kinds of food they eat. You may wish to refer to *Who Eats What Food?* to prompt studens during the brainstorming. Label one column "Eats Plants," another column "Eats Animals," and the third column "Eats Plants and Animals." Tell students that the term for animals that only eat plants is **herbivore.** Animals that eat other animals are called **carnivores.** Animals that eat both plants and animals are called **omnivores.** Label each column with the appropriate term. Have students record this information in their LiFE Logs.

Review the Module Question with students and ask them to reflect on it and record their thoughts in their LiFE Logs. *What have you learned so far? Have your ideas changed? What evidence do you have to support your new ideas?* Remind students that they will continue to learn more about the answer to the Module Question in Units 3, 4, and 5.

4. Discuss Feeding Relationships

Return to the list of organisms on the chart paper. Divide the class into five groups. Assign each group one of the organisms on the list. Give each group one index card and two different color markers. Have each group choose a recorder to label the card with the name of the group's organism and whether it is a producer or a consumer. Use one color marker for these labels.

As a class, invite students to discuss which types of consumer are included in the list.

What does this insect eat? What type of consumer is it? What does the frog eat? What kind of consumer is it? Follow this line of questioning for each consumer. If students disagree, ask them to cite evidence to support what they think. Bring the discussion to a close. Have each group recorder use the other color marker to write the food source on the group's index card.

5. Create a Food Chain

Invite a representative from each group to bring his or her index card and stand near the bulletin board. Tell students that they are going to make a visual model of a food chain that will show where each organism gets its food. Have the "producer" pin the plant index card on the board. *What eats the plant?* Pin a strand of yarn in a straight line leading from the plant card. Have the "insect" student pin the card at the end of the strand of yarn. *Which consumer eats the insect?* Pin another strand of yarn in a straight line from the insect card and continue forming the food chain (plant to insect to frog to snake to hawk). Use a different-colored strand of yarn for each link. Explain that this display demonstrates a food chain. It shows feeding relationships. Emphasize that a food chain only shows one source of food for each consumer. In an ecosystem, consumers may be part of several different food chains.

6. Conclude Unit 2

Engage students in a discussion of food chains. Point out that each organism is linked to the one before. *What would happen to our food chain if there were no frogs? What if there were no plants — what would the insect eat? If there were no plants, would anything happen to the hawk's food source?*

Return to the Unit Question: *If there were no plants, would humans have food?* After a brief class discussion, ask students to write two or three paragraphs in their LiFE Logs that answer this question in their own words. Guide their writing with the following questions — you may wish to write them on the board as a reference for students. *What have you learned that helps you answer this question? What evidence do you have to support your answer?*

Who Eats What Food?

HERBIVORES	CARNIVORES	OMNIVORES
Bighorn sheep	Ambush bugs	Bats
Cottontail rabbits	Ant lions	Humans
Cows	Assassin bugs	Moles
Deer mice	Falcons	Wild turkeys
Elk	Frogs	
Grasshoppers	Garter snakes	
Hares	Hawks	
Moose	King snakes	
Moths	Ladybugs	
Porcupines	Newts	
Squirrels	Owls	
	Racer snakes	
	Toads	
	Tree frogs	

Understanding Food Chains

Imagine a field or meadow ecosystem. In the summer the vegetation that grows here might include berries, wildflowers, and grasses. A young rabbit nibbles on the wildflowers, unaware of the fox nearby. The fox catches the rabbit and brings it back to its den, where its young are waiting. The fox kits eat the young rabbit. The next day the fox kits are playing in the grass near the den. An eagle flying overhead snatches one and carries it away to eat it. These events describe one food chain in this ecosystem. Food chains illustrate the path of food consumption from plants to animals. Arrows are used to show the direction of the energy flow; for example, an arrow would point from wildflowers to the rabbit. Another arrow would point from the rabbit to the fox. The last arrow in this food chain would point from the fox to the eagle.

It's important to remember that a food chain only shows one possible source of food for each animal. Most plants and animals are members of several different food chains. Another food chain in this meadow ecosystem might show a rabbit eating grass and the eagle eating the rabbit. A third food chain might show the kits eating the berries and the eagle eating a kit. Each example illustrates the transfer of energy and matter from one organism to another.

Note that food chains begin with plants, producers. The other organisms in the food chain are consumers, living organisms that consume other living things for food. All animals are consumers. In this lesson students are introduced to three different kinds of consumers: herbivores, or animals that only eat plants; carnivores, or animals that eat other animals; and omnivores, or animals that eat both plants and animals. In the next unit, students will continue to build their understanding of the flow of energy and matter through an ecosystem when they learn about other important members of an ecosystem: decomposers and scavengers.

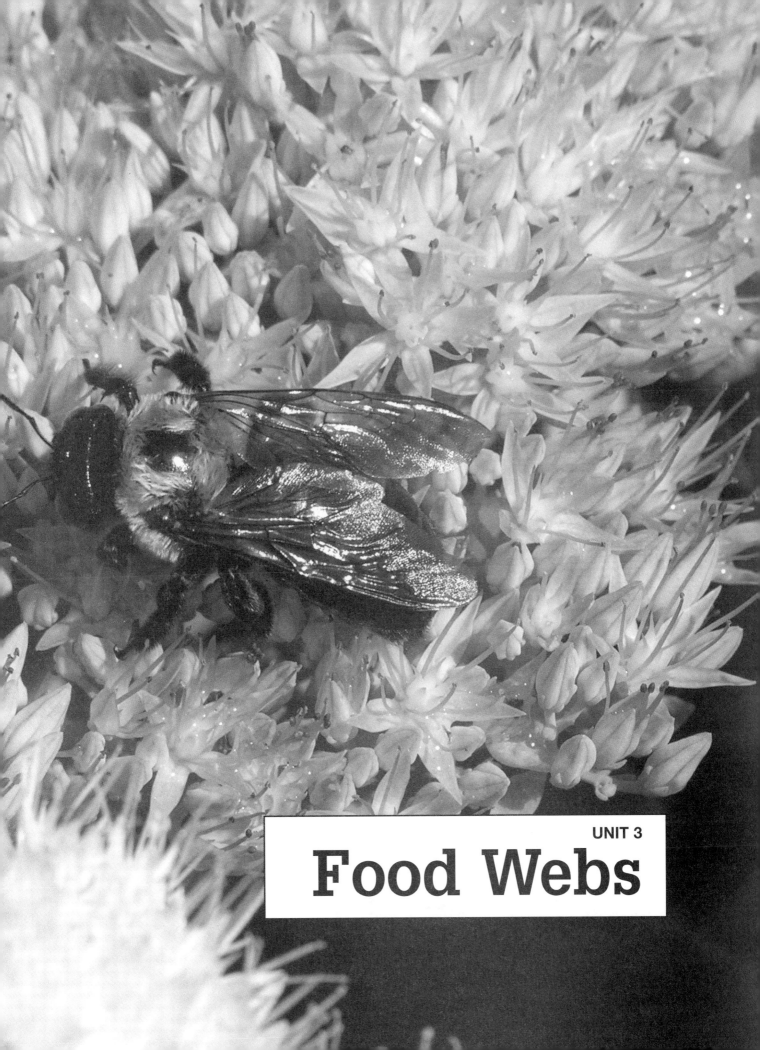

Food Webs

Nature's Decomposers

AIM

To understand nature's system for recycling nutrients.

SCIENTIFIC PROCESSES

• question, explore, research

OBJECTIVES

Students will be able to:

• discuss the role that scavengers, detritivores, and decomposers play in nature;

• describe the detritus food chain;

• discuss the importance of decomposition.

OVERVIEW

In this lesson, students begin to explore the Unit 3 Question, *How do components in nature interact with each other?* Through student readings, your class discovers that in nature there is no waste. Scavengers, detritivores, and decomposers consume dead plant and animal matter, scattered food particles, and animal excrement. Members of the detritus food chain are active, processing huge amounts of organic matter and releasing lots of energy, mostly as heat. Encourage your students to share their ideas about what they think happens to all of the organic "litter" in the natural world. You may discover that many of your students believe it "just rots," or "disappears." Some students may say that "bugs" are involved. Don't be surprised if the process of decomposition is not understood. What's important with this lesson is to find out what views, if any, students hold. This lesson helps prepare students to begin their hands-on investigation of decomposition in Lesson 10.

MATERIALS

For the teacher:
• *Decomposition* sample conversation
• *Making a Compost Bin* lesson resource
• Materials from *Making a Compost Bin* lesson resource
• *Setting Up the Compost Bin* lesson resource
• *LiFE Tips for Classroom Composting* lesson resource
• *Compost Bin Troubleshooting* lesson resource
• *Interactions in Nature* lesson resource
• *Detritus Food Chain* teacher note

For the class:
• Compost bin

For each student:
• *Recycling in Nature* student reading
• *Season of Plenty* student reading
• *Frost in the Air* student reading
• *Signs of Life* student reading
• LiFE Log

PROCEDURE

Before You Begin:

- Although you will be setting up the compost bin in Lesson 10, you will show students the bin at the end of this lesson. Please make or buy the bin for this lesson. See *Making a Compost Bin* lesson resource.

- Review the *Detritus Food Chain* teacher note.

- Review the *Setting Up the Compost Bin, LiFE Tips for Classroom Composting,* and *Compost Bin Troubleshooting* lesson resources.

- Review the *Interactions in Nature* lesson resource.

- Review the *Decomposition* sample conversation

- Make copies of the *Recycling in Nature, Season of Plenty, Frost in the Air,* and *Signs of Life* student readings to distribute to students.

- If you have not already done so, post the Module Question and the Unit 3 Question at the front of the class.

MODULE QUESTION

How does nature provide us with food?

UNIT QUESTION

How do components in nature interact with each other?

 QUESTIONING

1. Review the Module and Unit Questions

Introduce the Unit 3 Question. Briefly discuss that Unit 2 was all about plants and their role in nature, and that this unit moves onto other components of nature and how these interact with each other. Explain that in Unit 3 they will study the question *How do components in nature interact with each other?* If you have not

already done so, post the Unit 3 Question along with the Module Question and Unit 1 and 2 questions.

2. Summarize Unit 2

Review with students what they have learned about plants and animals. Remind them that they have been learning about how plants make food and how animals interact with plants. Review food chains and how matter and energy in food get passed along from plants to animals. Point out that most often when we imagine a food chain, we are thinking about one that includes green plants and animals that depend on these plants. Explain that sometimes the energy does not come from green plants, but instead comes from dead or decaying plants and animals. This type of food chain is called the detritus food chain.

Explain that students will investigate next what happens to all the plant and animal waste in nature, and what happens when plants and animals die.

3. Read about Waste in Nature

Explain that the detritus food chain introduces some new types of feeding relationships. Invite students to share some of their ideas about what happens to all the waste in nature. See the *Decomposition* sample conversation for an example of how this conversation might go in your class. *What happens to all the leaves after they fall off the trees? What happens when an animal in the woods or in a field dies? How about animal droppings or dead plants?* Accept all answers.

Remind students of some of the terms scientists use to describe the interactions in a food chain. *What can we learn from terms like "predator" or "prey"? What does the term "producer" tell us? What about "consumer"?* Explain that the organisms that make up a detritus food chain help release nutrients by breaking down dead and decaying material. Scientists categorize these organisms as decomposers, detritivores, and scavengers. Help students understand how terms that describe different kinds of interactions help scientists classify relationships in an ecosystem. Refer to the teacher note for more details about the detritus food chain. You may wish to begin a class list of different categories of relationships and add examples as you work through this unit.

SEARCHING

4. Introduce Decomposition

Remind students that in the **Searching** phase of QuESTA, they research a topic to learn more about it. Through their research, students learn what scientists already have found out about what happens to waste in nature. Have students work in small groups. Distribute the *Recycling in Nature* student reading to each student. After students have completed the reading and studied the illustration, give them several minutes to discuss what they have read in their small groups. *Does anyone have any new ideas about what happens to waste in nature?*

5. Read and Discuss Decomposition

Distribute the other student readings. Have students read about the changes that take place over time and study the illustrations. Use the *Interactions in Nature* lesson resource to guide their reading. After they have finished, give students several minutes to discuss with their group members what they have learned. Engage students in a class discussion based on their readings. *What have you learned? Have your ideas changed about what happens to waste in nature? Do you think that the decaying plants and animals decompose quickly? Why or why not?* Remind students to cite their evidence. Help students understand that time, temperature, and soil conditions all affect how quickly matter decomposes. You may wish to have students design

their own investigations of decomposition in your local area. Encourage students to think about the temperature, rainfall, decomposer community, soil type, and vegetation types where you live. Compare the conditions where you live to those depicted in the student readings. Invite students to discuss their ideas.

6. Introduce Compost Bin Project

Explain that in the next lesson the class will set up a compost bin so they can observe the process of decomposition themselves. Show students the compost bin and describe its features. Introduce students to the red wiggler worms that will be at work in the bin. Engage students in a discussion of what the worms need in order to live and grow. *What do living things need to survive and grow?* (air, water, food, shelter). *How will they get air?* Point to the holes on the side of the bin. Explain that the worms' food will include plant waste, coffee grounds, eggshells, and tea bags. Their shelter will be the compost bin filled with shredded newspaper. Worms need a dark, moist environment to survive. Demonstrate how to mist the newspaper to keep it moist. Point out the small holes in the bottom of the bin that allow any water that builds up to drain out. Place the lid on the bin to keep the worms' environment dark. Explain that this will be a long-term investigation. The class will observe the process of decomposition for the rest of the school year.

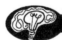

THEORIZING

7. LiFE Logs

Ask students to write one or two paragraphs in their own words that explain what it means when someone says there is no waste in nature.

Decomposition

This sample conversation in the **Questioning** phase of the QuESTA cycle will help you guide your students though a discussion that will allow them to think deeply and thoughtfully about the topic they are about to study. During the conversation, students may ask questions, think about what they already know, speculate on answers to questions, and wonder about what they are going to learn. This is a guide. Feel free to adjust your questioning to the needs of your class.

MS. M: We have already learned how plants make their own food using energy from the sun and how animals, including humans, depend on plants for food. Now we are going to learn about what happens to plants and animals after they die. *Have you ever wondered what happens to all the leaves that drop off the trees each fall?*

ANNA: When they are on the ground, people crunch them into the soil.

MS. M: Yes, good thought. *How about deep in the forest where there aren't any people?*

ANNA: Lots of bugs live in the woods. I wonder if bugs eat the leaves?

MS. M: *Do you think that there might be something that lives in soil that might eat them? How do you think we can find answers to our questions?*

ANNA: I know there are worms in the soil. We found some in my grandmother's garden.

MS. M: Yes, worms do live in the soil. *Do you think they might eat the soil?*

FRANCISCO: Well, worms and bugs need food to survive, so they must eat something. Maybe we could watch some worms and see if they eat leaves.

MS. M: Good idea! *What do you want to learn from watching worms eat? Where do you think the leaves go when the animals eat them?*

FRANCISCO: I wonder what happens to the leaves when they eat them? If worms are like us, they probably go to the bathroom — you know, they pee and poop.

HALEY: Yuck! I never want to touch soil again!

MS. M: I am glad you said that, because I bet everyone was thinking the same thing. Worm poop is not like human poop. Worms don't digest things the same way we do. Worm poop is called castings. Castings are very good for the soil. *Any idea why?*

JULIAN: Maybe something good in the leaves comes out in the worm castings.

MS. M: That's a good thought. Yes, the nutrients that were in the leaves are in the worm castings and end up in the soil. It's part of a cycle. We can learn more about this in our Reading for LiFE.

Continue the conversation to include a discussion of what happens when animals die.

Making a Compost Bin

Plastic or wooden? For indoor composting, either will do. The dimensions are the same, as is the placement of the holes on the sides and in the bottom. The advantage to using wooden bins is that they "breathe," which makes maintenance easier. However, wood is expensive and it is harder to make a wooden bin than to modify a plastic one. Unless you are a woodworker or know someone who is, try the plastic bin.

MATERIALS

For One Compost Bin

- Plastic bin (about 15"x24"x15"–18" high) with tightly fitting cover
- Fiberglass screening (about 2' square)
- White glue or glue gun
- Candle or gas burner

- Screwdriver
- Utility knife or drill
- Permanent marker
- 30" square piece of $1/2$" metal screening (for castings filter screen)
- Roll of duct tape

To Prepare the Bin

1. Heat a screwdriver with the gas burner or candle.

2. Poke 40–50 holes in the bottom of the bin. These small holes provide drainage if extra water builds up.

3. Heat a utility knife. Cut 6 holes, about 2"x3", on the sides near the top of the bin. Make 2 holes on the long sides, and one on each short side. If you don't have a utility knife, use a large drill bit — the kind used to make doorknob holes — to make several circular holes on each side. These holes in the side let air get into the bin.

4. Cover the holes on the side of the bin with the fiberglass screening. Glue the screen with white glue or a glue gun. Use ample glue to really make a seal at the edge of the screening.

5. (Optional) Use the permanent marker to number the inside walls of your compost bin, as shown at right. You can add food to one numbered section each week.

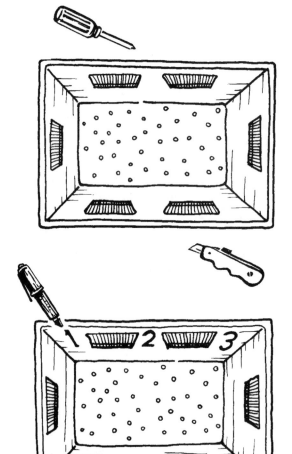

(continued on next page)

6. Fold duct tape around the edges of the 30" square metal screening. This screen will serve as the filter for the worm castings that you harvest.

Note: If you want to use a wooden bin, check with a local wine or liquor store. They often have wooden boxes that work well as compost bins. Some even come with lids that latch. If you prefer to purchase a compost bin, visit the National Gardening Association's Gardening with Kids online store (*www.kidsgardening.org*).

Purchase Red Wiggler Worms

You will need one pound of red wiggler worms for your box. Check for red wigglers at local gardening or composting facilities. You also can purchase them from the National Gardening Association's Gardening with Kids online store (*www.kidsgardening.org*).

Setting Up the Compost Bin

Location

Find a spot for your compost bin where the temperature range is 40°–85°F. Red wiggler worms thrive in temperatures that range from 55°–77°F. Be sure to keep the compost bin away from any heating unit. The worms will die if the compost gets too hot. If possible, keep a thermometer in the bin to monitor the temperature. The process of decomposition generates heat, so the compost will be warmer than the classroom.

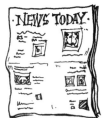

Compost Bin "Habitat"

Place lots of moist shredded paper in your compost bin to mimic a red wiggler's natural habitat of leaves, manure, or old compost piles. To shred the paper, fold two large sheets in quarters and tear lengthwise (with the grain of the paper) into 1/2", or thinner, strips. Have students help you shred enough newspaper to fill the entire compost bin. Shredded newspaper holds water well and is easy to keep fluffy so air can circulate. Air movement decreases the chance of odor. For best results add some dried, fallen leaves or garden mulch that has been in contact with soil.

Red Wiggler Worms

These worms are the primary decomposer in the compost bin. Bacteria and other microscopic organisms will live there as well, but they can't be seen with the naked eye. These worms are pretty resilient, which makes them ideal for classroom composting. If a little too much water is added or the bin attracts fruit flies, these worms most likely will be fine.

Food

Decomposers need food to live. Feed the worms your leftovers. You can add all the food at one time during the week, or you can add some every day or so. Either way is fine. Do what works best for you and your class. Remember to put the food scraps on top of the compost and below the bedding. If you saved the food scraps from Lesson 6 (*Celebrating Plant Parts*), plan to use these in the compost bin. See *LiFE Tips for Classroom Composting* on the next page for tips on what food to put in your compost bin.

Moisture

Water provides the moisture that worms need to survive. Monitor the moisture very carefully. If the compost bin gets too wet, the worms will crawl up the side to escape from the water. If it's too dry, they will die. Consider using a tray underneath the bin just in case any moisture leaks out.

Caring for Your Compost Bin during School Vacations

Add food and newspaper and give a healthy spray of water just before vacation and your bin will be fine for two to three weeks. Be sure to leave the bin in a place where it will not get too hot or too cold.

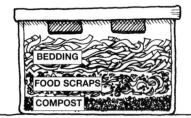

BEDDING

FOOD SCRAPS

COMPOST

LiFE Tips for Classroom Composting

Yes

- Raw vegetable trimmings
- Coffee grounds and filters
- Tea bags
- Finely crushed eggshells
- Used paper towels and napkins
- Trimmings from healthy house-plants and flowers
- Dried leaves or mulch that have some soil on them

If you are new to composting and want to make sure your compost bin does not develop odors or attract bugs, only add items from this list.

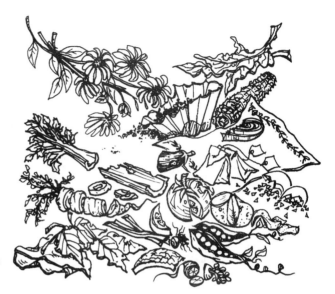

Maybe

- Raw fruit scraps
- Cooked vegetables and fruit

These foods can cause odors, create conditions where mold will grow, or attract bugs. If you microwave these foods for one minute on high, or freeze them, it will reduce the possibility of attracting bugs. Thaw before using.

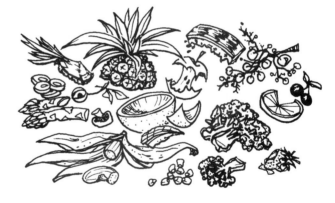

No

- Animal products
- Anything greasy
- Grains, beans, or breads
- Feces from dogs, cats, or birds
- Wood prunings

These items can cause odors and attract bugs and rodents.

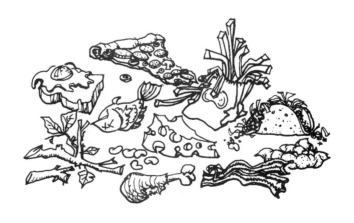

Compost Bin Troubleshooting

Has the level of the bedding dropped?

Shred more newspaper into a garbage can or other vessel, add water, mix well, and add this fresh, moistened newspaper to the top of the bin.

Are there dead worms?

Check to see if the bin is too hot or too cold. Bins kept next to a radiator may get very hot. If the worm population seems to be slowly decreasing, add food more often.

Is the bin too wet or too dry?

Worms crawling up the sides may mean the bin is too wet. Worms clumped together may mean it is too dry.

Are there lots of castings/compost at the bottom of the bin?

If yes, it is time to harvest.

Does the bin smell bad?

Stop adding fruit and vegetables and add more bedding, dried fallen leaves or mulch, and coffee grounds. When the odor is gone, resume adding scraps.

Is there mold in the bin?

Remove moldy food and bedding.

Are there fruit flies or other flying insects?

Stop adding fruit for a while and add some powdered limestone. Take the bin outside and open it for an hour or two to let the fruit flies or other insects fly away.

Are there reddish-brown mites?

If you see tiny, round-bodied, reddish-brown organisms with eight legs in your compost bin, they are mites. These particular mites like wet bins and can be quite a nuisance. If you find your compost bin has them, here are some things to do. Throw away the foods that the mites prefer — you can tell which ones because they will be covered with mites. Don't add any more of these particular foods for a while. For example, we've found that mites are attracted to bananas, so we don't add them anymore. Mites are attracted to slices of bread. To get rid of the mites, add slices of bread to the top of the compost pile and leave them overnight. Once the mites are on the bread, throw it away. Try to dry out the bin by leaving the lid off overnight, setting it out in the sun, or adding more bedding.

Interactions in Nature

Guiding Questions

Use the questions below to guide students in their readings for this lesson.

Recycling in Nature

Have students look at the illustration that accompanies the reading. Suggest that students make notes in their LiFE Logs about what they see in the drawing.

1. *What different kinds of food do you see in the drawing?*
2. *What different kinds of animals do you see?*
3. *What do this reading and illustration tell you about how animals in a field ecosystem get the energy they need to survive and grow?*
4. *What clues do you get about nutrients being recycled? What happens to the waste in the field?*

Season of Plenty

Have students look at the drawing and read the text beneath it. Have students add to their earlier notes.

1. *What are some of the ways that living things are interacting in this reading?*
2. *Are there interactions other than feeding? What is the bee doing?*
3. *Do you see any signs of interactions with nonliving things?*
4. *What happens when it rains?*

Frost in the Air

Have students look at the drawing and read the text beneath it. Have students add to their earlier notes.

1. *What are some of the nonliving parts of the field ecosystem at this time of year?*
2. *How do living and nonliving things interact in this illustration?*
3. *Why do some of the living things leave in fall?*
4. *What evidence do you have to support your thinking?*
5. *What can you learn about what happens to dead and decaying plants and animals?*

Signs of Life

Have students look at the drawing and read the text beneath it. Have students add to their earlier notes.

1. *What are some of the nonliving parts of the field ecosystem at this time of year?*
2. *How did nonliving things affect the field ecosystem in this reading?*
3. *What happens if there is no food to eat? Do all of the animals leave?*
4. *What evidence can you find that there will be new food sources?*
5. *Can you find evidence of nutrients being recycled?*

Detritus Food Chain

In Lesson 8 students learned about food chains, one of the ways that scientists can track the transfer of food energy and matter through an ecosystem. Producers make their own food through the process of photosynthesis. Consumers forage or hunt to find their food. But what happens to all the organic waste? What happens to the dead plants and animals? This organic debris, or detritus, is an important source of nutrients. With this lesson, we introduce some members of the detritus food chain — scavengers, detritivores, and decomposers. Scavengers, like crows, vultures, cockroaches, and bald eagles, eat dead plants and animals. They help break down dead organic materials into smaller pieces. Detritivores are multicellular organisms, like worms, insects, and nematodes, that mainly eat decomposed plants and/or animals. They break up or shred the organic matter that is their food. Decomposers, like fungi and bacteria, don't have mouths to ingest their food. Their food energy comes in the form of chemicals they absorb from decaying organic matter. The breakdown or decay of organic material is also called decomposition.

This lesson sets the stage for students to start contemplating how components in nature interact with each other. Students will begin to realize that interactions in an ecosystem are not limited to feeding relationships. The living components of an ecosystem not only interact with each other, they also interact with the physical and chemical components that make up an environment. An ecosystem can be as small as a drop of water or as large as, or larger than, a tropical rainforest. When you think about it, it's not surprising to hear that living organisms interact with nonliving components. Think about such processes as photosynthesis, respiration, and evaporation. There are also sunlight, temperature, moisture, and wind. All of these nonliving components are part of the environment.

The detritus food chain depicted in this lesson is based on an ecosystem based in the Northeast United States. If you live in a different climatic region, you may wish to have your students investigate decomposition in your region. You can use the **Interactions in Nature** lesson resource (on the previous page) as a guide. Challenge your students to conduct their own investigations using your school garden or other habitat as your study area. Have students use their LiFE Logs to record their observations of both the abiotic and biotic components over time.

How does this all connect to composting? As you prepare the classroom composting bin for Lesson 10, you will be creating an ecosystem with suitable environmental conditions for red worms to survive.

Name	Date

Recycling in Nature

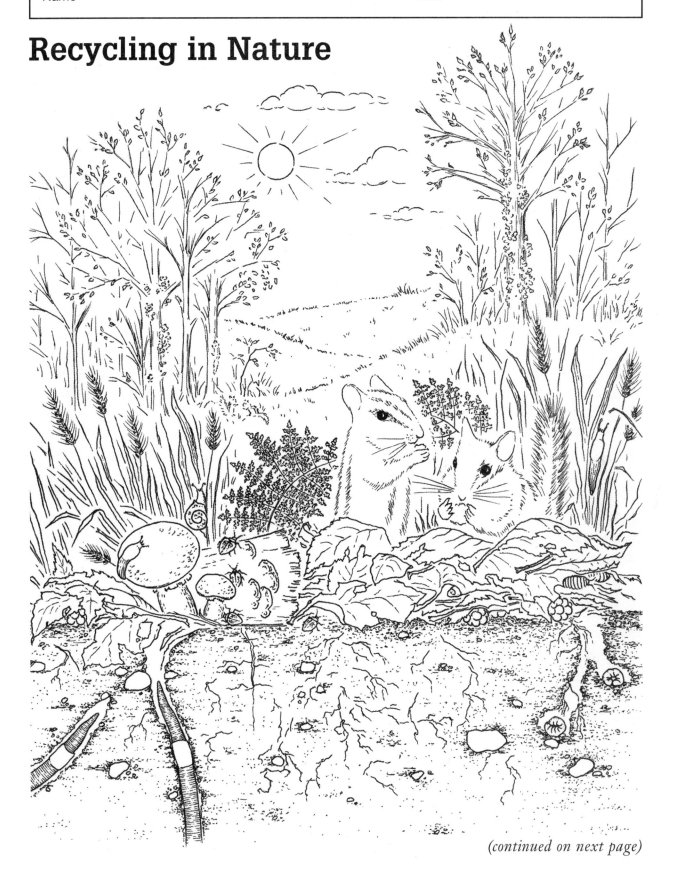

(continued on next page)

Name   Date

Recycling in Nature

There is no waste in nature. Have you ever heard anyone say that? What do you think it means? To find out, let's imagine a field in the spring. There are flowers poking up through the ground. Leaves cover the trees. Birds are building nests and laying eggs. Rabbits nibble on young plants. On an old stone wall you see some young chipmunks with their cheeks stuffed full of seeds. High in a tree, you spot an owl. Everywhere you look, you see signs of life. You visit the field every day for several months and you begin to notice that as time passes, things begin to change. You notice that the spring flowers are gone. You see a dead animal on the ground. As you look closer, you notice that part of the animal is missing. Did something eat it? Could it have been the owl? Next you see that insects are climbing on it. Are they eating it, too?

One day you see some plants that have died. You poke them with your toe and sow bugs and earwigs run for safety. You interrupted their meal. At your feet you see several dung beetles and you notice some animal droppings. The trees have lost their leaves. There is a thick layer of leaves under your feet. You lift up some leaves and see even more leaves in a thick mat. Some of them have been there for several years. You can tell because they have started to rot. They have something white growing on them. Maybe it's a kind of mold or fungus. You look over at an old tree stump at the edge of the field. It's covered with something that looks like mushrooms. The berry patch that once was full of juicy, ripe fruit has only a few half-eaten berries left. Some of the berries are on the ground. You look closer. They are covered with mold and are beginning to decay. Beneath your feet, deep in the soil, there is even more activity. Worms are burrowing tunnels. Old plant roots have broken off and are beginning to decay. Microscopic organisms are consuming the decaying plant material. What's happening?

You are observing another kind of energy transfer. In this energy transfer the organisms get their food energy from dead plants and animals and waste. They turn this organic matter into inorganic matter, like the nutrients found in soil. This process is called **decomposition.** How fast matter decomposes is affected by temperature, moisture, and the amount of oxygen in the soil. Eventually, all the organic matter on land that once was plant or animal is transformed into inorganic nutrients that become part of the soil. Now you understand what is meant by "There is no waste in nature."

Name   Date

Season of Plenty

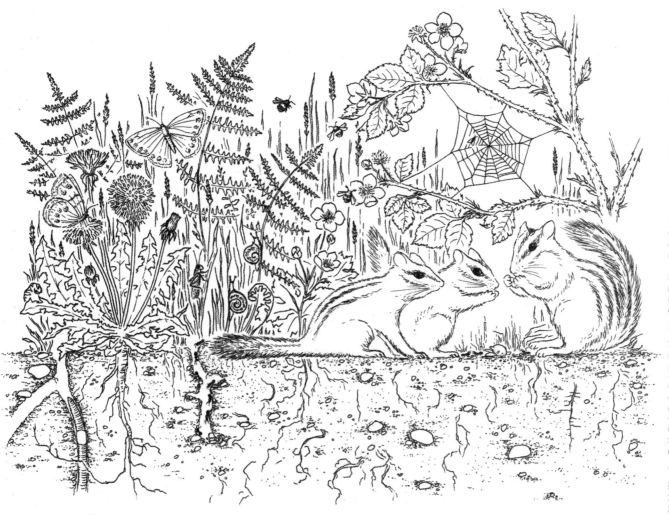

As spring slowly turns to summer, there are changes in the field. Spring rains and warmer temperatures help the flowers and grasses in the field grow. There will be lots of food for the animals that live here. Look closely and you will see that the air is alive with insects. Bees carry pollen from one flower to another. Butterflies sip nectar. Grasshoppers chomp on blades of grass. Snails creep along the ferns. At the edge of the field you see a spiderweb stretching between two branches of a berry bush. A fly is caught in the sticky web. Nearby, a chipmunk family nibbles on seeds. The ground is littered with food particles that they drop. You notice some movement. It's a long line of ants marching toward an anthill. They move quickly, carrying the bits of the seeds the chipmunks leave behind. One by one, they disappear into the anthill. Just beneath the surface, worms tunnel through the soil.

Name   Date

Frost in the Air

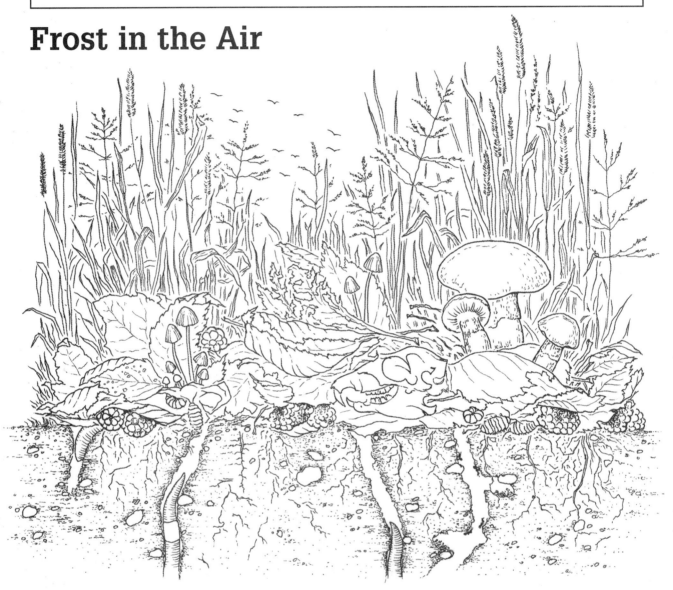

Fall is quickly turning to winter. Last night there was a heavy frost. As you look around you notice that there is very little green to be seen. Most of the flowers are dead. Their leaves are brown and wilted. The trees have lost most of their leaves. Some of them have blown into the field and crunch beneath your feet. You notice that the bees are gone. So are the butterflies. Their food sources are no longer here. Looking down, you see a few berries scattered on the ground. They are covered with mold. As you kick a pile of leaves, you see sow bugs scurrying away. You interrupted the process of decomposition. Your toe uncovered the skull of a small animal. All the flesh is gone. How many years has it been here? Overhead you see a flock of geese heading south for the winter. What has happened to all the life that filled the field in summer? Some animals, like the geese, migrate south and find new food sources there. Others, like the chipmunk, have stored food to eat when winter comes.

Name   Date

Signs of Life

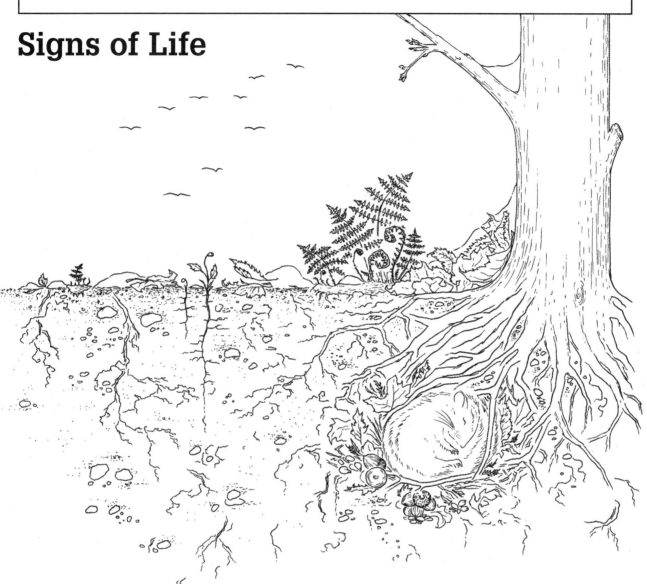

There was little activity in the field during the cold, harsh winter. There was not much food for the animals. Most of them migrated south or slept through the cold months. The freezing temperatures even slowed down decomposition. This will all start to change as the air warms and the soil begins to thaw. Soon the snow is almost gone. Only a few patches are left in the shade, protected from the warm sunlight. When you look down, you see early signs of spring. Seedlings begin to poke through the soil. The curled leaves of new ferns begin to show. Beneath the surface, safely tucked into its burrow, a chipmunk continues to nap. Tiny bursts of green appear on the tree branches. New leaves will soon cover the trees. Overhead you see migrating birds on their journeys north. Beneath your feet, microscopic organisms break down the wet, decaying leaf litter. What once was a bright green canopy of leaves is slowly being returned to the soil as nutrients.

Classroom Composting

OVERVIEW

Lesson 9 introduced students to the detritus food chain. In this lesson, they continue their investigations of decomposition by setting up a worm composting bin to gain hands-on experience with the decomposition process. The action in this lesson is setting up the compost bin. While you are doing this activity, be sure to make the purpose of the activity clear — the decomposition of food scraps. The resulting compost is rich in nutrients that can help grow more plants. Emphasize that this is nature's method of recycling. If you use the food scraps from Lesson 6, remind students that they got some of their energy by eating the salad. What they didn't eat, they fed to the worms. The worms used some of the energy. What the worms didn't digest, they excreted as castings. These castings are nutrient-rich and can be added to the soil and used to grow more plants to eat in another salad. In their LiFE Logs, students write what they think will happen in the compost bin.

AIM

To model decomposition in nature.

SCIENTIFIC PROCESSES

- question, gather data, research

OBJECTIVES

Students will be able to:

- identify what conditions are necessary for a healthy compost-bin environment;
- describe the process of decomposition that occurs in the compost bin;
- identify data they want to record on a composting data log;
- discuss how matter gets recycled through composting.

MATERIALS

For the teacher:
- *LiFE Tips for Classroom Composting* (p. 121) and *Compost Bin Troubleshooting* (p. 122) lesson resources
- *Setting Up the Compost Bin* lesson resource (p. 120)
- *Care and Feeding of a Compost Bin* lesson resource
- *Composting Bin Data Log* lesson resource
- *Worm Composting* teacher note

For the class:
- Compost bin (see p. 118 for details)
- Newspaper (see p. 120 for details)
- Spray bottle with water
- 1 pound red wiggler worms
- 1–2 pounds food scraps (see *LiFE Tips for Classroom Composting*, p. 121)

For each student:
- *All about Classroom Composting* student reading
- *Anatomy of a Worm* student reading
- LiFE Log

PROCEDURE

Before You Begin

- Review *Worm Composting* teacher note.

- Review *Setting Up the Compost Bin* lesson resource.

- Make copies of the *All about Classroom Composting* and *Anatomy of a Worm* student readings to distribute to students.

- Post copies of the lesson resources *LiFE Tips for Classroom Composting, Care and Feeding of a Compost Bin*, and *Compost Bin Troubleshooting* near the worm compost bin.

- If you have not already done so, post the Module Question and the Unit 3 Question at the front of the class.

MODULE QUESTION

How does nature provide us with food?

UNIT QUESTION

How do components in nature interact with each other?

 SEARCHING

1. Review the Module and Unit Questions

This lesson continues the class study of decomposition. In this lesson, students set up a compost bin to simulate decomposition in nature.

2. Research Composting and Worms

Distribute the two student readings *Classroom Composting* and *Anatomy of a Worm*. Have students read and discuss them in small groups.

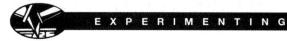 **EXPERIMENTING**

3. Set Up Model

Refer to the *Setting Up the Compost Bin* lesson resource to review the environmental conditions, food source, and inhabitants of the class composting bin. *If we looked outside, where could we find red wiggler worms?* (piles of leaves or manure or old compost piles) *What kind of food does a red wiggler eat?* (any organic matter) *What words can we use to describe the kind of habitat where red wigglers live?* (moist, dark places with ample food) *What kind of conditions does it need to survive?* (moisture, bedding, darkness, food).

If you have not already done so, shred enough newspaper to completely fill the compost bin. Pour two to three quarts of water over the top of the paper. Mix and fluff the paper until it is all evenly wet and is about as moist as a wrung-out sponge. Invite 4–5 student volunteers to help do this. Be careful not to add more water than the newspaper can absorb. If you do, the water may come out the drainage holes in the bottom. If you're using a plastic bin with a lid, you may wish to use it as a tray to catch any water that might leak out of the bottom. Be sure the newspaper is evenly wet, then add the red wiggler worms. Lift up some newspaper on one side of the bin and gently place half the worms on this side. Repeat for the other side. Next add the food scraps to begin the decomposition process. Always place the food under the moist newspaper. As you did with the worms, lift some newspaper out of one side of the bin and add about half the food. Repeat for the other side.

4. Make Predictions

Engage the class in a discussion about what they predict will happen in the bin. Through this discussion help students realize that there is only a little compost in the bin to start — the compost that came along with the worms. Over time, as students make observations, they will see more and more compost as the worms decompose the newspaper and food that has been put in the bin.

5. Develop Data Log

Review the *Compost Bin Data Log* lesson resource. Use this to guide students in a discussion of what data they want to gather and how they want to display that data to keep track of what happens in the compost bin. Decide who in the class will record what data on the log, to assure that it is always completed in a timely manner.

6. LiFE Logs

Have students predict what they think will happen in the compost bin. Remind them to include the information they are basing their predictions on.

Care and Feeding of a Compost Bin

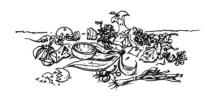

Food Scraps

Review *LiFE Tips for Classroom Composting.* If you are new to composting, start with the items listed in the "yes" list. As you get more comfortable you can begin adding fruit.

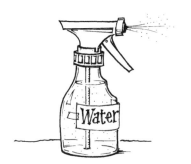

Water

Add water to your box every few days. Monitor the newspaper (bedding) on the top of the box. Spray water on the top layer every few days to keep the newspaper moist. Do not pour water on top. If you pour water onto the paper, most of it sinks to the bottom of the box. This makes the compost very thick and hard to harvest. *Note:* Wooden boxes dry out faster than plastic ones. Monitor the moisture level to determine how often to spray the newspaper.

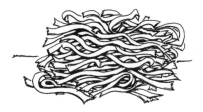

Bedding

To maintain a 4"–6" layer of bedding over the food, add shredded newspaper once every week or two. Moisten the newspaper in a large bucket or garbage can before you put it in the bin. This helps prevent water from accumulating at the bottom of the bin.

HARVESTING YOUR COMPOST

Harvest worm castings every 3–4 months to keep the worm population healthy. Use the castings as a top dressing on potted plants, flower beds, street-tree pits, or in gardens, or mix them with potting soil and use the mix as a seed-starting medium. It's important to harvest the castings, as they can become toxic to the worms over time. Follow these steps:

1. Do not add any food to the box for 2 weeks, so the worms get very hungry.

2. Move the compost with worms to one side of the bin.

3. Place the old bedding and some fresh bedding on the empty side. Bury food scraps in the bedding. Every few days add water only to the side of the bin with the bedding and food. Within 2–4 weeks the worms will migrate to the new food and the finished castings can be removed.

4. The castings on the top of the pile will dry out first and can be removed. Take out the castings by handfuls until you start to see worms. In a few days you will be able to take out a few more handfuls.

5. Filter the finished compost through the worm-castings filter screen. Anything that doesn't go through the screen gets put back into the bin.

6. As you filter, keep an eye out for worms and gently return them to the compost bin.

7. After removing the finished compost, add additional bedding and food to the bin.

Compost Bin Data Log

Develop a log to keep track of what happens with the class compost bin. Brainstorm with students a list of all the data they would like to collect. Here is an example.

Date bin was set up: _____

Number of worms (or pounds of worms) added to bin: _____

Number of students adding food scraps on a regular basis: _____

Date	Weight of Food Added	Type of Food Added	Amount of Water Added	Notes

Worm Composting

Making a compost bin, populating it with red wiggler worms, and then having to care for and feed those worms may seem like a lot of work. You already have so much to do, who needs one more long-term project?

It's true, vermicomposting in the classroom is a project and worms don't take care of themselves. That being said, we've found that most teachers who tried it were delighted. Why? The students' enthusiasm was one major factor. Students loved learning about worms and taking care of them, and in the process, they had a real-life experience with decomposition. What better way to help students learn about recycling organic waste and participating in a natural cycle? Teachers also found that once they started composting, it really didn't take as much time as they'd feared. There are "short cuts" that you'll learn along the way. Our instructions are to guide you — you don't need to follow them to the letter. You'll find that worms don't have to be fed every week. Harvesting the castings may be a task you turn over to a student volunteer who does it once a week and harvests just a section of the bin at a time. Compost however it works for you.

We simply urge you to try it. We're convinced that once you start, you'll get hooked and will want to learn even more about composting.

Mary Appelhof's *Worms Eat My Garbage* is an excellent resource for anyone experimenting with vermicomposting.

Worm-Handling Tips

Many students will ask to hold a worm. This is fine as long as they handle the worms with care. Remind students that the worms are not pets. They play an important role in the decomposition cycle. They perform an important function. Without scavengers, decomposers, and detritivores, we would be buried in organic waste.

To hold a worm, gently pick it up with one hand — be sure not to squeeze too hard — and place it on the palm of the other hand. Sometimes a worm may move very quickly and almost "jump" in your hand. At other times a worm may be so still you wonder if it is alive. Remember: worms are light sensitive. Use your hand to shade them from the light.

Finally, worms are not solitary creatures. They live in a community. If a student ever asks to take home one worm as a pet, gently explain that removing one worm from the bin would not be good for the worm. Even if the student promises to take really good care of the worm, point out that worms live in a community and need other worms.

Remind your students that the purpose of having the compost bin is to learn about the process of decomposition by modeling what happens in nature. Their task as scientists is to observe and record what happens in the compost bin.

Name	Date

All about Classroom Composting

The compost worms' natural habitat is piles of leaves, manure piles, and old compost piles. Compost worms, also called red worms or red wigglers, are different from the earthworms you usually find in the ground.

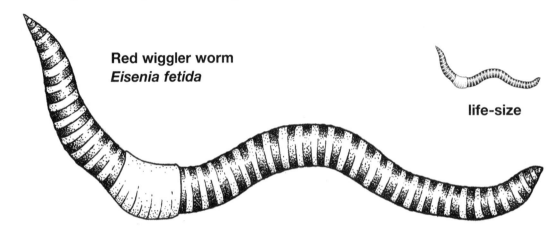

Red wiggler worm
Eisenia fetida

life-size

Environmental Conditions

Like all living things, worms grow and live best when the conditions are just right. Worms like the dark. Sunshine dries worms out and can kill them. Keep the compost bin dark. Worms like a moist environment, but not a wet one. Red wigglers can live in a wide range of temperatures. They eat, grow, reproduce, and survive best in temperatures between 55°–77°F. A worm can live for a few weeks to one year. The number of worms, and how long they live, depends on how healthful the environment is where they are living.

Bedding

In their natural habitat, red wigglers live under lots of moist bedding, like leaves. However, for an indoor compost bin, black-and-white newspaper makes a great substitute. The paper holds moisture well and is easy to keep fluffy. Be sure to keep at least 6" of bedding on top of the food at all times.

Moisture

Use a spray bottle to keep the bedding moist. You may need to add a little water every few days. Do not overwater! Given too much water the worms will die.

Food

Worms eat plant material. You can feed them tea bags, coffee grounds, eggshells, vegetable scraps (such as corn husks and corn cobs, peppers, carrots, tomatoes, lettuce, potatoes), and fruit. It is important for the food in the compost bin to be broken into small pieces. Plan to add food to the compost bin every week.

Name

Date

Anatomy of a Worm

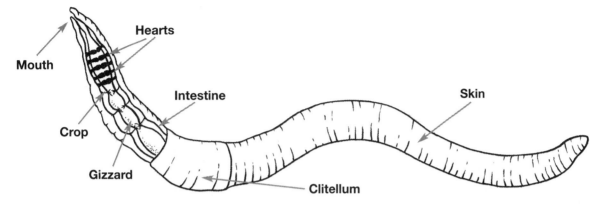

Hearts

Mouth

Intestine

Skin

Crop

Gizzard

Clitellum

Eisenia fetida is the scientific name for red wigglers or red worms. These worms are used for indoor compost bins. Read on to learn more about these amazing decomposers.

Look at the drawing. Notice that the worm has five **"hearts."** These hearts actually are five pairs of large blood vessels. Blood travels through the body and brings oxygen to all the parts of the worm. Worms need moist environments so they can breathe. But if the environment is too wet, the worms will move to dryer spots. Have you ever seen worms on top of the ground during a rainstorm? They are trying to get to a dryer place. It can't be too dry, though. If it is, the worms will dry out and die.

Red wigglers reproduce quickly, so there are always plenty of worms. Find the **clitellum.** This band hardens and forms a cocoon that the worm slides over its head. Each cocoon can hold up to 20 fertilized eggs. After about three weeks, the eggs hatch.

Red wiggler worms eat food scraps and other plant material. Look at the drawing and find the worm's mouth. The food travels from the **mouth** to the **crop,** where it is broken down into smaller pieces. Sometimes food is stored in the crop. Next the food passes into the **gizzard,** where it is broken down into even smaller pieces. The gizzard is made of strong muscles that act like teeth. Sand in the gizzard helps grind the food. Finally, the food passes into the **intestine,** where digestion is completed. The worm gets nutrients and energy from the digested food. The worm excretes the undigested food as waste. This waste, also called **castings,** is what makes up compost.

DID YOU KNOW ... ?

Earthworms

- have taste buds
- breathe through their skin
- hear by vibrations

Webs of Interactions

AIM

To explore ecosystem interactions.

SCIENTIFIC PROCESSES

• model, infer, discuss

OBJECTIVES

Students will be able to:

• identify interactions between organisms and the physical environment;

• describe in words and through a web diagram how some components in nature interact with each other;

• use scientific reasoning to justify their web.

OVERVIEW

This is the final lesson in the unit that explores how components in nature interact with each other. In this lesson, students draw on the knowledge they have gained in the module and create a web that illustrates how the biotic and abiotic components of an ecosystem interact with each other. Students study a scientific illustration of a field ecosystem and record their observations in their LiFE Logs. Using these observations, as well as reviewing what they have learned about interactions in prior lessons, students work in small groups to create their web of interactions. Each group presents its work to the class. At the end of each presentation, there is a short period for students to discuss or debate the group's findings. For homework, students infer the effect that humans and human activities might have on a field ecosystem.

MATERIALS

For the teacher:
• *Who Eats What Food?* lesson resource (p. 111)
• *Understanding Food Chains* teacher note (p. 112)
• *Detritus Food Chain* teacher note (p. 124)
• *Field Ecosystem Interactions* lesson resource
• *Biotic and Abiotic Interactions* lesson resource
• *Learning from Nature* teacher note

For each group of 3–5 students:
• 2 sheets of chart paper
• Markers

For each student:
• *Recycling in Nature, Season of Plenty, Frost in the Air,* and *Signs of Life* student readings (pp. 125–129)
• *Ecosystem Interactions* activity sheet
• *Modeling Interactions* activity sheet
• LiFE Log

PROCEDURE

Before You Begin:

- Review the *Understanding Food Chains, Detritus Food Chain,* and *Learning from Nature* teacher notes and the *Field Ecosystem Interactions* and *Biotic and Abiotic Interactions* lesson resources.

- Make copies of the *Ecosystem Interactions* and the *Modeling Interactions* activity sheets to distribute to students.

- You may wish to make copies of the *Field Ecosystem Interactions, Who Eats What Food,* and *Biotic and Abiotic Interactions* lesson resources for student groups to share.

- If you have not already done so, post the Module Question and the Unit 3 Question at the front of the class.

MODULE QUESTION

How does nature provide us with food?

UNIT QUESTION

How do components in nature interact with each other?

 THEORIZING

1. Review the Module and Unit Questions

Explain that in this lesson students will be pulling together all they have already learned about the Module Question and summarizing it to answer the Unit 3 Question.

2. Summarize Unit 3

Review with students what they have learned about roles that different organisms play in an ecosystem. You may wish to allow students about five minutes to review their LiFE Log notes from earlier lessons, as well as their student readings. Remind students that they have been learning about feeding relationships and how energy flows through an ecosystem. *What are some of the different types of feeding relationships that we've been discussing?* (producer, consumer, herbivore, carnivore, omnivore, decomposer, scavenger, detritivore) *Who can explain why there is no waste in nature? What happens to dead and decaying plants and animals?* If necessary, review food chains and how matter and energy in food get passed along from plants to animals.

3. Discuss Food Webs

Remind students of the diagrams they made in Lesson 8. *How many sources of food per animal did our food chains show?* (one source of food per animal) *In this lesson, we're going to explore more complex interdependence. Can anyone tell me what a food web is?* Explain that food webs show the feeding relationships among many species in a community. *All of these interactions are examples of who eats what. Can anyone think of other kinds of interactions that take place in an ecosystem that make it possible for an organism to survive?* Tell students that next the class will discuss some of the basic needs of plants and animals.

4. Discuss Biotic and Abiotic Factors

You may wish to have students review the student readings from Lesson 9 before you begin this discussion. *What are some of the living, or **biotic,** factors in a field ecosystem? Can you think of some of the nonliving, or **abiotic,** factors in a field ecosystem?* If students need prompts, encourage them to think about what plants need to make food. *What other conditions affect plant and animal life?* (weather, temperature, water, etc.) *Can you think of an animal or a plant and some of the conditions it needs to be able to survive and grow in an ecosystem? If these conditions don't exist, what happens to the plant or animal? Think about what you learned in Lesson 9 and life in the field ecosystem at different times of the year. What are the conditions that change in the spring, summer, fall, and winter? Do these conditions affect the plant and animal life in the field? How?*

Distribute the *Ecosystem Interactions* activity sheet. If students are struggling with the concept of biotic and abiotic interactions, you may wish to review these terms as a class and identify several of the biotic and abiotic elements that are shown in the illustration.

5. Introduce Ecosystem Interactions Project

Distribute the *Modeling Interactions* activity sheet to each student. Review the activity instructions with the class. Have students work in small groups. Give each group two sheets of chart paper and markers. You may wish to give students a copy of the *Field Ecosystem Interactions, Who Eats What Food?,* and *Biotic and Abiotic Interactions* lesson resources. Tell students they can refer to any of their resources from Lessons 8 and 9 as well as their LiFE Logs to help them with this project.

6. Present Web Diagrams

Explain that an important part of being a scientist is sharing work with other scientists, which is often done at scientific meetings. *We are going to have a science-sharing meeting now to learn about the webs of interactions developed by each group.* Allow each student group about five minutes to present its web diagram. You may wish to have student groups select one person in the group to be the presenter. Post each group's diagram at the front of the room.

Invite the class to ask the presenting group clarifying questions or to debate any of the information that is presented. Once all of the groups have presented, have a class discussion that compares and contrasts the various diagrams. Use this discussion to solidify students' understanding of the interdependence of nature. Be sure to add or clarify any concepts that students do not discuss.

The goal of this discussion is to review the role of biotic and abiotic factors and how these factors interact with each other. Work with students to draw conclusions about the importance of interactions within ecosystems and how these interactions allow the organisms to survive. You may wish to have groups remove one abiotic or biotic element from their interactions web and discuss what they think might happen to life in the field ecosystem. Monitor the length and depth of this discussion to gauge how well your students understand these concepts.

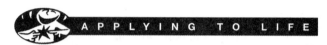 APPLYING TO LIFE

7. LiFE Logs Homework

Have students write a few paragraphs in their LiFE Logs that discuss how humans and human activities might affect ecosystem interactions. Prompt students by having them think about what might happen if humans picked all the berries in the field or mowed the grasses growing there. Have students conclude their writing by thinking about the abiotic factors in the environment that humans need to survive and grow.

Field Ecosystem Interactions

This page includes details of some of the biotic (living) and abiotic (nonliving) components shown in this lesson's field ecosystem illustration, as well as a list of some of the interactions. Use this resource, as well as *Biotic and Abiotic Interactions,* to help guide your students in their web-diagram activity.

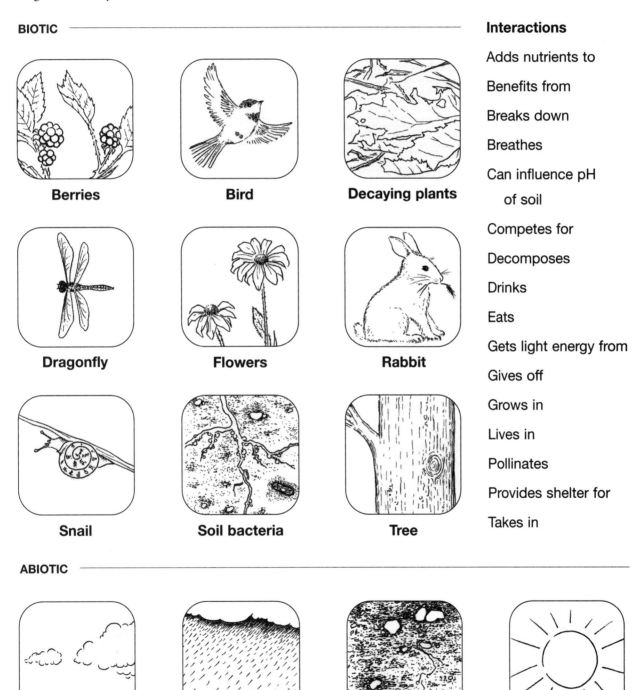

BIOTIC

Berries

Bird

Decaying plants

Dragonfly

Flowers

Rabbit

Snail

Soil bacteria

Tree

Interactions

Adds nutrients to

Benefits from

Breaks down

Breathes

Can influence pH
   of soil

Competes for

Decomposes

Drinks

Eats

Gets light energy from

Gives off

Grows in

Lives in

Pollinates

Provides shelter for

Takes in

ABIOTIC

Air

Rain

Soil

Sun

Biotic and Abiotic Interactions

An ecosystem, such as the field ecosystem illustrated throughout this unit, is made up of physical and biological components. These components interact with each other. If one component changes, the others might be affected. For example, if there is little rain during the summer and the berry bushes don't produce much fruit, this food source will be reduced. In turn, this might reduce the size of the berry-eating animal population. If there are fewer berry-eating animals, this will affect the animals that depend on berry-eating animals as their food source, and so forth. In short, lack of sufficient rain, a physical component, can set off a series of chain reactions, or interactions. The opposite can also occur. Sufficient rain can result in a bumper crop of berries, which can lead to an increase in berry-eating animals, as well as an increase in their predator populations.

The example below shows some basic biotic and abiotic interactions. Energy from the sun goes to plants. Food energy from plants goes to consumers. Plants take in and give off atmospheric gases and water. Consumers take in and give off atmospheric gases. Detritivores consume dead and decaying organic matter from consumers and producers. Detritivores give off nutrients to the soil and gases to the atmosphere. Plants take in nutrients and water from the soil.

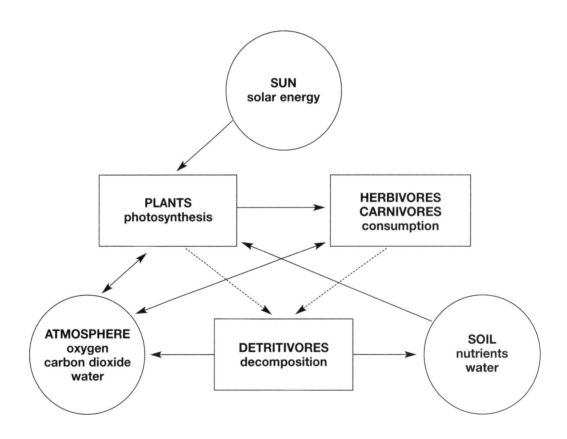

Learning from Nature

This lesson pulls together what students have learned thus far in the module. It also sets the stage for the Unit 4 Question, *How do we interact with nature to meet our food needs?* Unit 4 introduces students to farmers and farming practices. Agriculture means humans are managing the landscape. To be a successful farmer means understanding how the natural world works, particularly what plants and animals need in order to grow and thrive. Essentially, with agriculture, humans manipulate the environment to create favorable conditions for crops to thrive. Farmers create an ecosystem of producers (plant crops) and consumers (animals).

As you begin this lesson, check for student understanding of an ecosystem. Make sure that students understand that ecosystems are made up of a community of living organisms and the community's physical environment. These biotic and abiotic components continuously interact with each other. Be sure students grasp that changes in one component often cause changes in another. For example, in a temperate climate, a seasonal change from summer to fall brings with it a change in temperature. As a result, plants may die, food sources change, and some animal populations hibernate while others migrate to warmer climates. If they did not, they would run the risk of dying. A drought that causes plants to die also removes a food source and causes changes in the consumer populations. Birds that nest in trees will move elsewhere if the trees are cut down. Be sure to stress that interactions in an ecosystem may be beneficial or they may be harmful.

Name	Date

Ecosystem Interactions

In this activity, you are going to be a scientist studying a field ecosystem. Look closely at the illustration of a field ecosystem and imagine you are studying the **biotic,** or living, and **abiotic,** or nonliving, elements in it. Use the questions on the next page to guide your observations.

(continued on next page)

Name   Date

Ecosystem Interactions

To survive in an ecosystem, plants and animals interact with each other and with non-living things. Study the illustration carefully, think about what you see, and keep field notes in your LiFE Log. As you examine the drawing, think about how the biotic and abiotic elements interact in the ecosystem.

1. How many different kinds of plants do you see? Circle them or list them in your LiFE Log.

2. How many different kinds of animals do you see? Circle them or list them in your LiFE Log.

3. Look for evidence of abiotic elements that affect how plants and animals grow and survive. Think about such things as light, temperature, water, wind, soil, gases in the air, and so forth. List them in your LiFE Log.

4. Look at the drawing and think about interactions that take place between plants and animals. Describe at least three interactions in your LiFE Log. *Hint:* Sometimes animals use plants for shelter and sometimes animals pollinate plants.

5. Look at the drawing and think about interactions that take place between plants and some of the abiotic elements in the ecosystem. Describe at least three in your LiFE Logs. *Hint:* What do plants need to grow and survive?

6. Look at the drawing and think about interactions that take place between animals and some of the abiotic elements in the ecosystem. Describe at least three in your LiFE Logs. *Hint:* Animals drink water. Where does it come from? Animals take in oxygen. Where does it come from?

Name   Date

Modeling Interactions

You and your group members will make a chart or diagram on chart paper that shows some of the web of interactions that you found when you studied the illustration of a field ecosystem. Use the information on this page to help you with your work.

1. Decide as a group how you want to draw your web of interactions. You can make a list and draw lines between the different biotic and abiotic elements to show the interactions. Or you can make a sketch of the field ecosystem and draw in lines to show the interactions.

2. Draw lines between the elements to show where there is an interaction. Use arrows to show the direction of the interaction. For example, to show an interaction between a chipmunk and air, you would draw an arrow from the air to the chipmunk, with the arrow pointing toward the chipmunk. The arrow shows that the chipmunk takes in air. Write what kind of interaction takes place on top of the line. For example:

breathes
Air - - - - - - - - - - - ➤ Chipmunk

3. Give your web of interactions a title. Write the title across the top of the chart paper.

Growing Food
©2007 Teachers College Columbia University

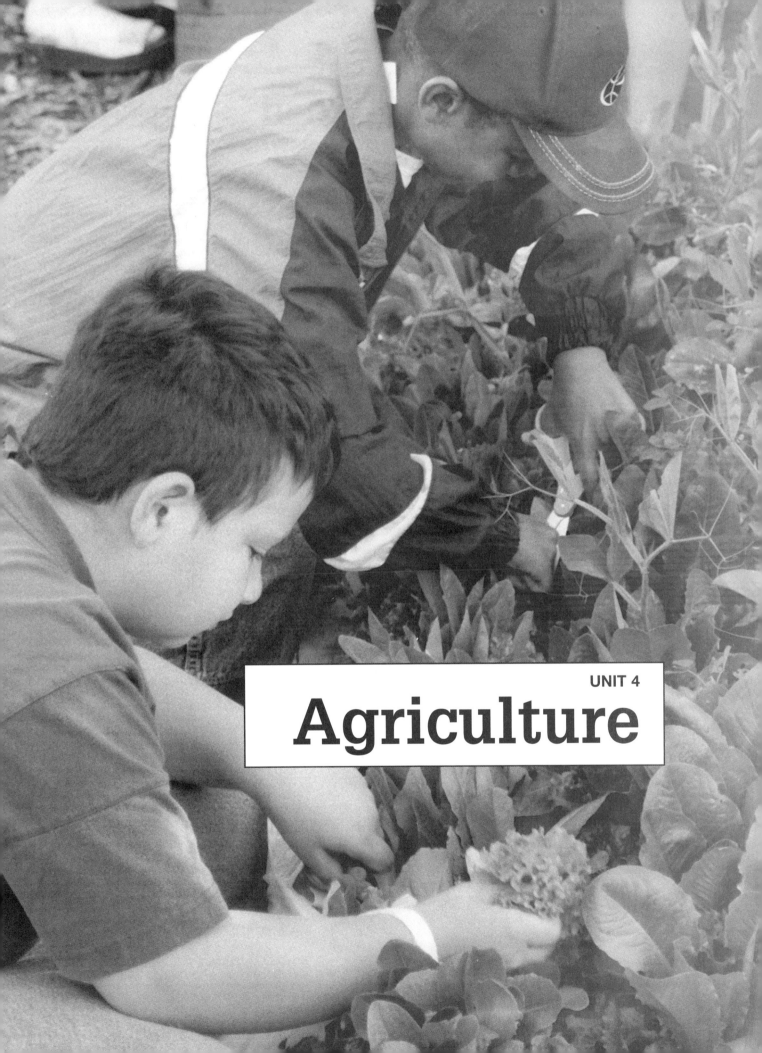

UNIT 4
Agriculture

No Farmers, No Food

AIM

To recognize and value the role of farmers in growing the plants and raising the animals that humans eat.

SCIENTIFIC PROCESSES

• contemplate, speculate, construct knowledge

OBJECTIVES

Students will be able to:

• discuss the role of farmers in growing the plants and raising the animals we eat;

• value farmers for the role they play in our food system;

• appreciate how our lives would be different without farmers.

OVERVIEW

Thus far, students have been exploring how nature provides us with food. They've learned about the difference between plants (producers) and animals (consumers) and they've gained an understanding of photosynthesis and the flow of energy through a simple food web. Their studies have focused on the natural world. Now students begin to explore the Unit 4 Question, *How do we interact with nature to meet our food needs?* In investigating this question, students begin their study of the human-managed landscape, the designed world of agriculture. More specifically, students begin to recognize the role humans play in producing the foods we like to eat. Through analyzing some whole and processed foods, students gain an understanding that farmers grow or raise much of the food we eat. Using their LiFE Logs they decide what kinds of plants and animals they would like to grow if they were farmers, and then draw a picture and write a paragraph to describe this.

MATERIALS

For the teacher:
• *From Farm to Store* sample conversation
• *Introducing the Food System* teacher note

For the class:
• Chart paper (at least 5 sheets)
• Markers
• 1 apple
• *Apple Products Analysis* lesson resource

For each student:
• *Apple-Filled Cereal Bar Analysis* activity sheet
• LiFE Log

PROCEDURE

Before You Begin:

- Review the *Introducing the Food System* teacher note and the *From Farm to Store* sample conversation.

- Prepare the chart paper. Write, *Why do we need farmers?* on the top of the first sheet of chart paper; *How would your life be different without farmers?* on top of the second sheet; *Apple* on top of the third sheet; the ingredient list for apple-flavored yogurt as a list down the left side of the fourth sheet; and the ingredient list for apple-filled cereal bars as a list down the left side of the fifth sheet. These lists are on the *Apple Products Analysis* lesson resource. Do not record the information in the key on the chart. Use it to guide the student discussion. Post these sheets of chart paper in the front of the room.

- Make copies of the *Apple-Filled Cereal Bar Analysis* activity sheet for each student.

- Lesson 13 is a planting activity. If you have not already done so, order, or purchase locally, seeds, planters, soil, and compost. Refer to the *Getting Started with Classroom Crops* lesson resource in Lesson 13 for indoor gardening and seed selection tips.

- If you have not already done so, post the Module Question and the Unit 4 Question at the front of the class.

MODULE QUESTION

How does nature provide us with food?

UNIT QUESTION

How do we interact with nature to meet our food needs?

 QUESTIONING

1. Introduce Unit 4 Question

Remind students that in Units 2 and 3 they learned about the role of nature in food production. Review the first three Unit Questions with students. Introduce the Unit 4 Question and explain that in this unit students will be learning about the role that humans play in producing our food.

2. Appreciate Farmers

Did you grow the food that you ate today? If you didn't, who did? Why do we need farmers? How would your life be different if there were no farmers? Record some of your students' responses on the chart paper. Accept all answers. You will add to this list later on in the lesson.

Even though we don't often think about it, farmers grow the plants or raise the animals we eat. Just about every food is made from ingredients that started out as a plant or came from an animal. If we did not have farmers to grow our food, we would need to spend a large amount of our time growing it ourselves.

 THEORIZING

3. Analyze Foods

Hold up an apple and ask students to share what they know about how apples grow. Record their ideas on the left side of the chart paper labeled *Apple*. Tell students where you purchased the apple. Next, ask them to speculate about the steps it took to grow this apple and get it to the store or farmers' market where you bought it. If the apple came from a farmers' market, you may know quite a bit about where and how it was grown. However, if it was purchased at a supermarket, you may know very little about its "history." Record the students' ideas on the right side of the chart paper.

Show students the ingredient list for apple-flavored yogurt. Engage students in a discussion of all the types of plants and animals farmers had to grow or raise to make this yogurt. Record their ideas on the chart paper.

Have students think about the fruit-flavored yogurt they buy in stores. Based on what they learned about the apple-flavored yogurt, ask them to consider the origins and production of their favorite fruit-flavored yogurt. Use these questions to guide student thinking. *What do we already know about how fruit-flavored yogurt is made? Which ingredients were grown or raised by farmers? Where do you think the ingredients were mixed together to make yogurt? How did they get there? How were they mixed to make yogurt? How did the yogurt get to the market?* Encourage students to brainstorm and share all their ideas. Accept all answers and summarize what is said on the chart paper.

Distribute the *Apple-Filled Cereal Bar Analysis* activity sheet to each student. Have students work in small groups. Let student groups choose an ingredient from the cereal bar ingredient list or assign each group one of the ingredients. After students have completed the activity sheet, have them record their responses on the chart paper. Have students speculate about the origins and manufacturing of the cereal bar, as they did for the apple-flavored yogurt.

4. Discuss Farming as Part of the Designed World

Through this discussion help students understand that the world we live in is very different from the natural world. In the previous units we examined nature and the interdependence of life in the natural world. The focus of this unit is the human-designed world of agriculture.

Think about the world we live in today. *Do we eat whatever plants and animals are available and close by? Why do you eat some foods but not others? Do humans have likes and dislikes?* In today's world, most of us can be very selective about the foods we eat. Our food choices are influenced by our cultural heritage, our age, our gender, our friends, our family, and where we live. However, we have not always been so selective.

Early in human history, people were hunters and gatherers and depended on nature for their survival. Then this began to change. Based on archaeological evidence found in the Near East, we know that about 11,000 years ago humans began to domesticate plants, goats, and sheep. There is also evidence that between 5,000 and 10,000 years ago there were agricultural systems in China, North America, South America, and Africa. By about 2,000 years ago most human populations depended upon agriculture.

Today, our world is shaped by our actions. We intentionally design and manage the landscape to serve our needs. Imagine what the landscape looked like before there was large-scale farming. *What was the United States like when the pioneers traveled west? What kinds of changes do you think took place when humans began to farm the land?* We disrupt nature's web of life to selectively grow crops and raise animals that suit our tastes. This means there are fewer resources and less space for other living organisms, like plants, bacteria, mammals, insects, and the rest of the animal kingdom, to live and reproduce.

5. Introduce Food Systems

What if there were no farmers? Would our lives be different? How would we get the food we need to survive? Have any of you ever grown any of your own food on a farm or in a garden? Have students share their experiences. Encourage discussion of how long it takes to grow vegetables from seed. Through this discussion, help students appreciate how much time and effort it takes to produce enough plants and animals for humans to eat.

Agriculture brought with it changes in society. Help students make the connection between what they are learning about farming in this lesson and what they are learning about human history in social studies. *What are some ways that agriculture changed society? What would it mean if only some people were responsible for growing the food for everyone? Would other people be able to do different kinds of work? Do you think it might change how people lived?* Accept all answers. Point out that people can live in towns and cities because we have a food system that makes it possible. A simple way to describe a food system is getting food from the field to the table. However, a food system has many systems within it. For example, there are systems for growing food on the farm, and systems for preserving, processing, transporting, and packaging food.

The foods analyzed earlier in this lesson give examples of how our food system works. Even though we do not often think about our food system, it makes it possible for us to have a lifestyle in which we do not have to spend much of our time producing our own food.

See the sample conversation at the end of this lesson for an example of how this conversation might go in your class.

Return to the lists on the chart paper of initial ideas about *Why do we need farmers?* and *Would your life be different if there were no farmers?* Ask students for new ideas they would like to add to the list. Throughout this unit we will learn more about these topics.

6. LiFE Logs

Have students write a paragraph that begins with: "If I were a farmer, I would grow these kinds of plants and animals because. . ." Ask students to include as many details as they can and have them draw a picture of their farm. Remind students to include any questions they have about farms.

From Farm to Store

> This sample conversation in the **Questioning** phase of the QuESTA cycle will help you guide your students through a conversation that will allow them to think deeply and thoughtfully about the topic they are about to study. During the conversation, students may ask questions, think about what they already know, speculate on answers to questions, and wonder about what they are going to learn. This is a guide. Feel free to adjust your questioning to the needs of your class.

MR. R: *Now that some of you have shared experiences growing food, who can tell me something that happens to food between the farm and the store?*

MARIA: Food usually comes in a box or a container. They have to put food into these somewhere — I think it's in a factory.

MR. R: *Anything else?*

LENNY: Some foods, like the yogurt and cereal bar we talked about, have lots of ingredients that get mixed together.

MR. R: Right. This is called processing. And, as Maria just pointed out, food is usually packaged and processed in factories. *Who else has something to add?*

MAX: Food also has to get to the store. Sometimes I see trucks delivering food to the store.

MR. R: Good, food has to be transported. Food is also preserved, which means doing things to it that will keep it from going bad. To summarize, we have farmers who grow plants and raise animals for our food. Between the time food leaves the farm and arrives at the store it is processed, preserved, packaged, and transported. All of these steps for getting food from the farm to our tables are part of the food system. *What would our lives be like without our food system?*

TYRA: We would have to spend lots of time growing our food.

MR. R: Yes, you are right, growing and cooking all of our own food would take lots more time. Adults would do much of this work, but probably you would help, too.

ANGEL: To grow our own food we would have to plan ahead. It would take a lot of planning to make sure that we would have enough food. Now, we can walk into a store, decide what we want, and get it any time we want.

MR. R: Growing and cooking all of our own food would take lots of planning. *How else would our lives be different?*

ROSANNA: Farms need a lot of space for the plants and animals to grow. I don't think we could live in a city with houses close together and tall apartment buildings if we had to grow our own food.

MR. R: Good, now let's go back to our charts and see if we can add to our ideas about why we need farmers and how our lives would be different without farmers.

Apple Products Analysis

APPLE-FLAVORED YOGURT

Ingredient List

Milk
Sugar
Apple purée
Cinnamon
Nutmeg
Cornstarch
Live active cultures

Key

Milk — cow
Sugar — sugar cane or sugar beet plant
Apple purée — apple tree
Cinnamon — cinnamon tree
Nutmeg — nutmeg tree
Cornstarch — corn plant
Live active cultures — "good" bacteria

APPLE-FILLED CEREAL BAR

Ingredient List

Apples
Wheat flour
Oats
Nonfat dry milk
Pineapple juice
Pear juice
Sunflower oil
Corn syrup
Soy lecithin
Cinnamon
Baking powder
Salt

Key

Apples — apple tree
Wheat flour — wheat plant
Oats — oat plant
Nonfat dry milk — cow
Pineapple juice — pineapple plant
Pear juice — pear tree
Sunflower oil — sunflower
Corn syrup — corn plant
Soy lecithin — soybean plant
Cinnamon — cinnamon tree
Baking powder — acid, base, and filler
 (usually corn starch)
Salt — ocean

Introducing the Food System

Even though you eat food every day, you probably don't stop to think about how food gets from where it was grown or raised to where you bought it. Stop for a minute and think about the system or the steps that food goes through before it reaches you. Parts of the food system can include:

Preserving Food

Food preservation can be chemical or physical. Physical methods include drying, canning, or freezing. These methods take away the air (canning), the water (drying), or the warm temperature (freezing) that microorganisms need to grow. Chemical methods for preserving food include adding sugar, salt, vinegar, or other chemicals that create an environment too toxic for microorganisms to survive in.

Processing Food

This refers to changing a food's characteristics or properties. Food can be processed a small amount, a medium amount, or a large amount. Single foods can be processed a small amount, which may be done to make the food easier to eat, change its taste, or make it a more useful ingredient in a recipe. Some examples of processing single foods are making applesauce from apples; removing the bran from brown rice to make white rice; grinding wheat berries to make flour; whipping heavy cream to make whipped cream; grinding peanuts to make peanut butter; adding cultures to milk to make yogurt; and cutting carrots to make carrot sticks.

When several ingredients are mixed together, they are processed a medium amount. Most of the individual ingredients are usually still recognizable. Some examples are canned soup, dried soup, frozen dinners, and peanut-butter-and-jelly sandwiches.

When many ingredients are combined, they are processed a large amount. Most of the individual ingredients are no longer recognizable. Examples include cake, cookies, and cold cereals.

Many of the foods that are available in supermarkets are called "processed food products." This often means food that was made in a factory, and is made up of several ingredients.

Packaging Food

This step of the food system involves protecting food with a barrier to guard it from the outside. Typically, food packages are made from cardboard, plastic, glass, or metal.

Transporting Food

This step involves moving food from a farm to other places. On its journey from a farm to your table, food may stop at factories, warehouses, and stores. Food can be transported by truck, boat, train, or plane.

Name	Date

Apple-Filled Cereal Bar Analysis

Pick an ingredient from the list your teacher posted at the front of the room. Think carefully about the ingredient. You may want to search for more information in reference books or on the Internet. Write your answers below.

1. Name of ingredient _____

2. Is this ingredient from a plant or animal? _____

3. Think about the ingredient you are analyzing. Do you know what part of the world it grows in? *Hint:* If it is a plant, what growing conditions does it need to survive? Is it a tropical plant? If it is an animal, does it live on a farm or a ranch? Speculate where you think it may come from and why you think this is so.

_____

_____

4. Describe how you think the ingredient was turned into part of the cereal bar. *Hint:* How does a pear become pear juice?

_____

_____

_____

5. Where was the cereal bar made?_____

6. How did the cereal bar get to the market?

_____

_____

_____

Classroom Crops

AIM

To plant and care for vegetables and herbs from seed to harvest.

SCIENTIFIC PROCESSES

- contemplate, discover, contrast, investigate, implement

OBJECTIVES

Students will be able to:

- describe how to care for plants they want to grow and harvest;

- contrast the needs of different plants;

- apply the knowledge they have acquired as they care for their plants.

OVERVIEW

Through planting and caring for vegetables and herbs from seed to harvest, students continue to increase their understanding of nature's system for producing food and build their appreciation of the work farmers do to produce our food. Through researching information on the "seed packets" provided in this lesson, as well as the actual packets of seeds the class will grow, students determine how to grow and care for different kinds of plants. Using the information they have gathered, students plant their crops. Before planting the seeds, students compare and contrast the similarities and differences in the planting and growing needs of their classroom crops. During this long-term gardening project, students keep journals to document their experiences. In their LiFE Logs, students describe what they imagine it will be like to grow classroom crops.

MATERIALS

For the teacher:
- *Getting Started with Classroom Crops* lesson resource
- *Caring for Your Crops* lesson resource
- Chart paper
- Markers

For the class:
- 5 planters, 24"–36" long
- Soil
- Compost
- Seeds
- Watering can
- Masking tape
- (Optional) Wooden plant markers

For each student:
- Student readings from Lesson 6 (pp. 81–87)
- *Arugula* student reading
- *Basil* student reading
- *Borage* student reading
- *Chives* student reading
- *Cilantro* student reading
- *Cucumber* student reading
- *Dill* student reading
- *Onion* student reading
- *Parsley* student reading
- *Pepper* student reading
- *Radish* student reading
- *Tomato* student reading
- *Plant Information Table* activity sheet
- LiFE Log

PROCEDURE

Before You Begin:

- Review the *Getting Started with Classroom Crops* and *Caring for Your Crops* lesson resources.

- Fill each planter with a mixture of soil and compost (1 part compost to 2 parts soil).

- Make copies of the seed packet student readings to distribute to each student. Review the basic care needs outlined on the seed-packet student readings and the packets of seeds for your classroom crops.

- Divide the class into five groups, one group for each planter.

- If you have not already done so, post the Module Question and the Unit 4 Question at the front of the class.

MODULE QUESTION

How does nature provide us with food?

UNIT QUESTION

How do we interact with nature to meet our food needs?

 QUESTIONING

1. Review Module and Unit Questions

Remind students of the Module Question. Explain that with this lesson the class will begin a long-term project to further investigate the Unit 4 Question. We will plant vegetable and herb seeds to have an experience of growing crops in our classroom.

2. Discuss Growing Crops in the Classroom

Tell students that farmers grow crops in large outdoor fields. Since we don't have large fields for our project, we are going to grow our crops inside our classroom. *What is different about what farmers do compared to what we are going to do? What is similar?* Briefly have students share some thoughts. Explain that growing food is exciting no matter where you grow it. Create enthusiasm and excitement about the idea of planting seeds, watching for them to poke through the soil, nurturing them as they grow, and finally harvesting the mature plants to eat.

 SEARCHING

3. Explore the Needs of Different Plants

Explain that before farmers plant their seeds, they learn as much as they can about how to grow and care for the plants. The class will do the same. Have students look at the plant illustrations on the student readings. Engage students in a discussion of what they see in the illustrations. Point out that the drawings show the entire plant in both the above- and below-ground environments where the plant lives. Briefly review what students learned in Lesson 6 (*Celebrating Plant Parts*). Remind students that when they made their salad they learned that we eat different parts of different plants. *Look at the drawings of the plants we are being introduced to in this lesson — what parts of these plants do we eat?* We eat the roots of the radish; the leaves of the arugula, basil, borage, chives, cilantro, dill, and parsley; the flowers of the chives and borage; and the fruit of the cucumber, pepper, and tomato.

Review the information in the student readings and on the packets of seeds you are going to plant. Use this information to complete the *Plant Information Table* activity sheet. You may choose to write the information on the *Plant Information Table* on chart paper to post in your classroom.

Based on what you learned about the plants' needs and the number of different types of plants you are growing, decide which seeds to plant in each of the five planters.

EXPERIMENTING

4. Plant

Remind students to follow the planting instructions from the *Plant Information Table* when they plant the seeds.

Label each planter with the type of seed and the date the seeds were planted. Write this information on masking tape and stick it on the side of the planter. For planters with several types of seeds, you may prefer to write the plant names and dates on wooden plant markers and place them in the soil to indicate where the seeds were planted. Place all the planters in a sunny place in the classroom.

5. Create a Plan to Care for the Plants

Have each group select a person to be responsible for the basic care of each planter. Responsibilities can include watering, monitoring the amount of light, turning the planter when the plants grow toward the light, adding compost, thinning the seedlings if there are too many, etc. You may choose to assign students designated jobs for all the classroom crops (watering, turning, etc.), or you may prefer to have groups of students provide all the care for individual planters.

Record the basic care plan on chart paper and post it in a prominent place in the classroom.

6. Construct Classroom Crop Logs

Explain that students will use their LiFE Logs throughout this project to record their observations. Have the students designate a particular section of their LiFE Log (for example, the last 20 pages) as their Classroom Crop Log.

Tell students that every day, or every few days, they will observe the plants and record their observations in their Classroom Crop Log. Keeping a log is an important part of the learning process in this activity. By observing the plants and recording their observations, students have the opportunity to see how the plants change over time. Reviewing their notes also lets students reflect on how they take care of the plants. Be sure to set aside enough classroom time for students to make detailed plant observations.

Brainstorm with students a list of what kinds of information they might record (examples: how many seeds have germinated, when the seedlings develop their first set of "true" leaves, the number of leaves on the plants, the shape of the leaves, the direction the leaves are facing, and so forth). Have students record the height of the plants on a weekly basis.

 THEORIZING

7. Contrast the Care Needs of the Various Plants

Explain that farmers are keenly aware of the different needs of the crops they grow. Ask students to review the *Plant Information Table* and highlight some of the differences among the different classroom crops in terms of their need for light, water, and space. Tell students that really understanding what plants need to grow will help ensure that the class has a successful gardening experience with a bountiful harvest.

 APPLYING TO LIFE

8. LiFE Logs

Ask students to write a poem or a short paragraph that describes what they think it will be like to be classroom farmers over the next several months.

Getting Started with Classroom Crops

If you are new to gardening or have limited space in your classroom, start small. Herbs grow quickly and are ready to be harvested as soon as the plant is large enough to spare a few leaves. While vegetables generally take longer to grow to harvest, they are well worth the wait. The plants we have included in this lesson are all crops that typically grow successfully in classrooms. Look for plant varieties that grow well in container gardens in your region to increase your success. If you have a school garden or would like to start one, you can do this project in the garden. The more often the students visit the garden, the more they will fully appreciate how plants grow.

If you live in a warm climate and your school has the space, think about growing your crops outdoors. If you do set up a garden, make sure students still have ample opportunity to care for and investigate their plants and record their observations in their LiFE Logs.

Choosing Seeds

If you'd like some personal assistance in selecting which plants to grow, consider a trip to your local garden center or florist. The staff can offer suggestions on seeds that will be most successful for an indoor environment. Garden-center staff can help with decisions about selecting planters, soil, and compost. The garden center may also offer delivery service. Typically, each seed packet contains more seeds than you'll need. If other classes in your school are using LiFE, consider sharing your resources.

Many companies have online catalogs. For example, the National Gardening Association (NGA) has extensive resources available on its Web site (*www.kidsgardening.org*), including kits and materials specifically developed for classroom gardening. Burpee (*www.burpee.com*) is another online source.

Selecting Planters

Planters work well. We've even had success growing and harvesting tomatoes and peppers in our window boxes. Of course, large plants will do better if they are transplanted into larger containers that give the plants' roots more space. Any type of container will work. We reuse our planters from year to year. Just remember to clean them out thoroughly to prevent the growth of unwanted microorganisms.

LiFE advocates "community" gardening. Therefore we use planters so the entire class tends the garden rather than having individual students growing their own plants. Group gardening promotes a sense of community. In our experience, using single containers promotes competition.

Preparing the Soil

Purchase soil for indoor planting rather than bringing in soil from the outdoors, which may introduce unwanted pests. For natural fertilizer, add 1 part compost to 2 parts soil. Once the plants have started to grow, sprinkle more compost on top of the soil. When you water, the nutrients in the compost will "drip" into the soil.

Spread newspaper to catch any soil that spills when you fill the planters. Use the soil spills to top off the planter.

Caring for Your Crops

Watering Needs

Make certain your planters have drainage holes in the bottom. Be sure to use something under the planter to catch any water that drains out. Follow the watering directions on the seed packets. Some plants need more water than others. Be sure to water your classroom crops on Fridays to keep them moist all weekend long.

Available Light

Your classroom crops need as much light as you can give them. Put your planters in the sunniest location possible. If you can, move them outside during the day. Plants grow toward the light, so be sure to turn them frequently to ensure even growth. If the plants get "leggy," you'll know they need more light.

Growing Temperature

For seedlings, 60°–70°F is the ideal temperature. If it's too hot, the plants grow too quickly. This makes the cell wall thin and the plants weak. In extreme cases, weak cell walls will keep the plants from standing upright. While a windowsill is a logical spot for your seedlings, if there is a radiator near the window, it may make it too hot. Try to strike a balance between a sunny place and a spot that's not too hot for your plants.

Space to Grow

Plants need enough space to grow. If they are too close together, they compete for resources — light, water, and nutrients. The plants can even get entangled both above and below the soil. If your plants are crowded, you'll need to thin them out. This can be sad for you and your students. However, it's better to have fewer healthy plants than many plants competing to stay alive. Refer to the guidelines on your seed packets.

School Vacations

During school vacations, consider taking the classroom crops home. If this isn't possible, water the plants well before you leave for vacation. Another method is to create a "drip irrigation" system. Fill plastic drink bottles with water and insert the bottle mouth into the soil. The water will slowly drip out of the bottle and into the soil. Check to see if a member of the custodial staff will be at school during vacation. If so, ask a custodian to water the plants while you are away. If your vacation is during the winter, check to see what the classroom temperature will be. If there is a chance the room will be too cold for the plants, you can create a makeshift greenhouse by loosely covering the planters with transparent dry-cleaning bags.

Name   Date

ARUGULA

Eruca vesicaria

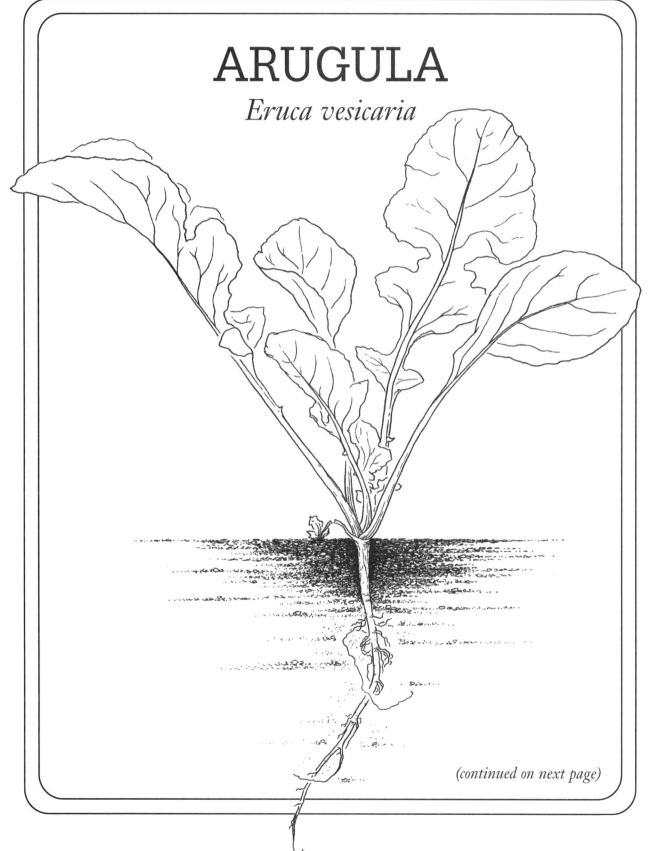

(continued on next page)

Name   Date

ARUGULA
Eruca vesicaria

ANNUAL VEGETABLE
Arugula is an example of one of the kinds of greens found in a salad mix called mesclun. These salad blends often have a wide variety of shapes, colors, and textures. Some other greens that might be included in a mesclun salad mix packet are: Tango, Royal Oak Leaf, Red Salad Bowl, Black Seeded Simpson, and Red Sails.

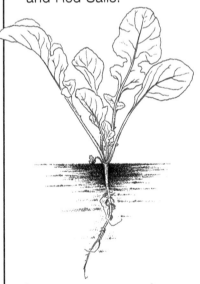

GROWING

Sow seeds after the last heavy frost. Arugula, like lettuce, is a cool-weather vegetable. It is best to grow arugula in early spring or fall. Plant seeds every 2", covering firmly with soil. Thin plants to about 6" apart when they have 2 or 3 leaves. Arugula needs regular watering.

HARVESTING

When plants are 3" tall, thin your plantings. Use these in your salads. As plants get taller, pick outside leaves or cut a section about 1/2" above the soil.

COOKING

Mix with other greens to give salad an interesting flavor. You can try any kind of dressing. A simple oil-and-vinegar dressing is delicious. Or, cook briefly in olive oil with garlic and serve with pasta and grated cheese.

Start seeds in the Northeast	Days to germination	Days to harvest	Planting depth	Plant spacing	Preserve by
March–April & July–August	7–10	40–60	1/4"	6"	Fresh use only

Growing Food
©2007 Teachers College Columbia University

BECOMING FOOD SCIENTISTS : PLANTS : FOOD WEBS : **AGRICULTURE** : MAKING CHOICES

Name   Date

BASIL

Ocimum basilicum

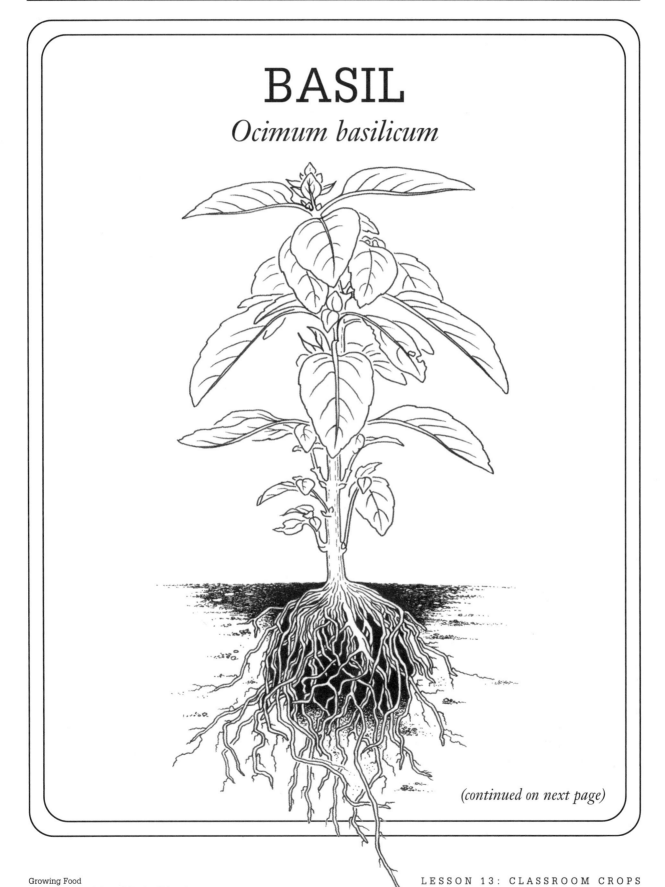

(continued on next page)

Name	Date

BECOMING FOOD SCIENTISTS : PLANTS : FOOD WEBS : **AGRICULTURE** : MAKING CHOICES

BASIL
Ocimum basilicum

ANNUAL HERB

The leaves of this herb have a spicy flavor and a fragrant aroma. Basil is a member of the mint family, and a favorite ingredient in Italian cooking. It is a great plant to grow in a sunny window in your home or classroom.

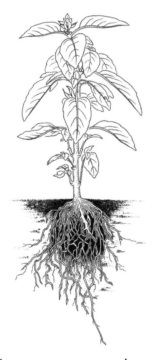

GROWING

Start seeds indoors in seed-starting mix 6 weeks before planting outdoors. Or plant directly outside in full sun after danger of frost is over and ground is warm. Grows best in rows 12" apart. Within each row, thin or transplant plants to 10" apart when they are 3" tall. Basil grows well in planters at least 8" deep. Basil has the fullest flavor when the plant is grown in full sunlight.

HARVESTING

To harvest, pinch off whole sections of the plant. This makes the plant bushy and keeps flowers from forming. Basil gets a bitter taste once flowers form. Pick basil early in the morning for fresh use.

COOKING

Use basil leaves fresh on sliced tomatoes, in pesto sauce, or cooked in stir-fries or in sauces. Take fresh basil and snip it into crushed tomatoes. Add sautéed garlic, onions, and mushrooms. Simmer about 15 minutes before serving over pasta or chicken.

Start seeds in the Northeast	Days to germination	Planting depth	Plant spacing	Plant height	Preserve by
April–July	5–10	1/4"	10"	18"–24"	Drying & freezing

Name   Date

BORAGE
Borago officinalis

(continued on next page)

Name   Date

BORAGE
Borago officinalis

ANNUAL HERB

This plant has clusters of blue flowers and a mild cucumber flavor. Both the leaves and the flowers are edible. Bees love borage. Borage is native to the Mediterranean. It is also a hardy, fast-growing plant that is quite easy to grow but requires a large area in the garden in order to thrive.

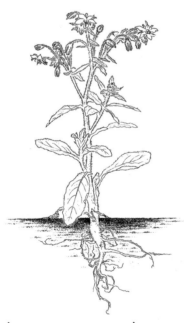

GROWING

Start seeds indoors in seed-starting mix 6 weeks before last frost. Or after all danger of frost, sow seeds in a place that gets lots of sun. Cover with 1/8" of soil. Thin plants to 12" apart when they are 2" tall. Plant borage in and around your vegetable garden to attract bees and help pollination of cucumbers, cantaloupe, eggplant, peppers, squash, pumpkins, and watermelon.

HARVESTING

Pick leaves or flowers anytime after plants are about 8" tall. The more you pick, the bushier the plant will get.

COOKING

Chop young leaves and use them in salads, or cook the leaves like spinach. Add the edible flowers to salads or use them for a garnish. Freeze 1 borage flower in each section of an ice-cube tray, then add the ice cubes to your favorite drink. You can also candy the flowers to decorate cakes and ice cream.

Start seeds in the Northeast	Days to germination	Planting depth	Plant spacing	Plant height	Preserve by
April–June	7–14	1/4"	12"	15"–24"	Fresh use only

Name

Date

BECOMING FOOD SCIENTISTS : PLANTS : FOOD WEBS : **AGRICULTURE** : MAKING CHOICES

CHIVES
Allium schoenoprasum

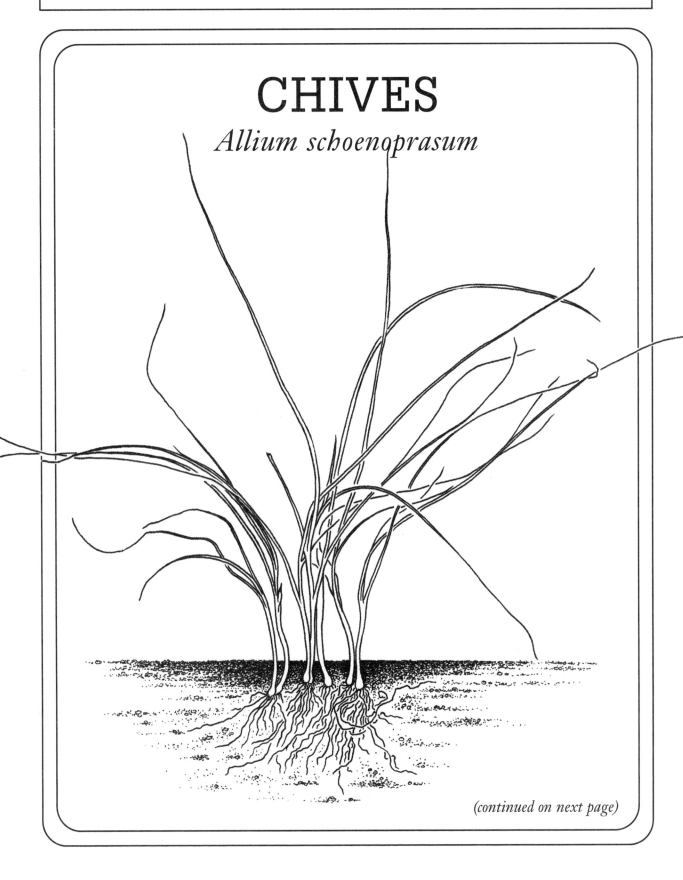

(continued on next page)

Name   Date

CHIVES
Allium schoenoprasum

PERENNIAL HERB
The hollow, thin leaves have a delicate flavor and taste like very mild onions. The purple flowers are also edible. Chives are well loved all over the world. They are native to Europe and Asia, and are one of the easiest herbs to grow.

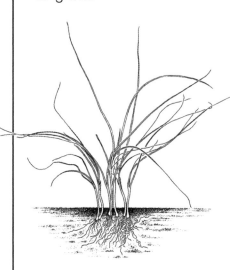

GROWING

Start seeds indoors in seed-starting mix 6 weeks before planting outdoors. Or sow seeds in the early spring as soon as the soil can be worked. Chives prefer a sunny location in rich, well-drained soil. They grow best in rows 12" apart. Thin plants to 6" apart when they are 2" tall. Or plant in a pot with good drainage. In winter, sink the pot into the ground to winter over.

HARVESTING

Begin harvesting about 6 weeks after you plant the seeds. Use scissors to snip chives off at the base of the plant. This pruning encourages new growth. Harvest the leaves the day you want to use them.

COOKING

Use chives fresh anywhere you might use onions. Chopped chives are delicious in salads, soups, and omelettes. The flowers are edible in salads or as a garnish. Chives are most tasty fresh but can be dried and sprinkled over baked potatoes or casseroles.

Start seeds in the Northeast	Days to germination	Planting depth	Plant spacing	Plant height	Preserve by
April–August	15–21	1/4"	6"	8"–14"	Drying or freezing

Name   Date

BECOMING FOOD SCIENTISTS : PLANTS : FOOD WEBS : **AGRICULTURE** : MAKING CHOICES

CILANTRO

Coriandrum sativum

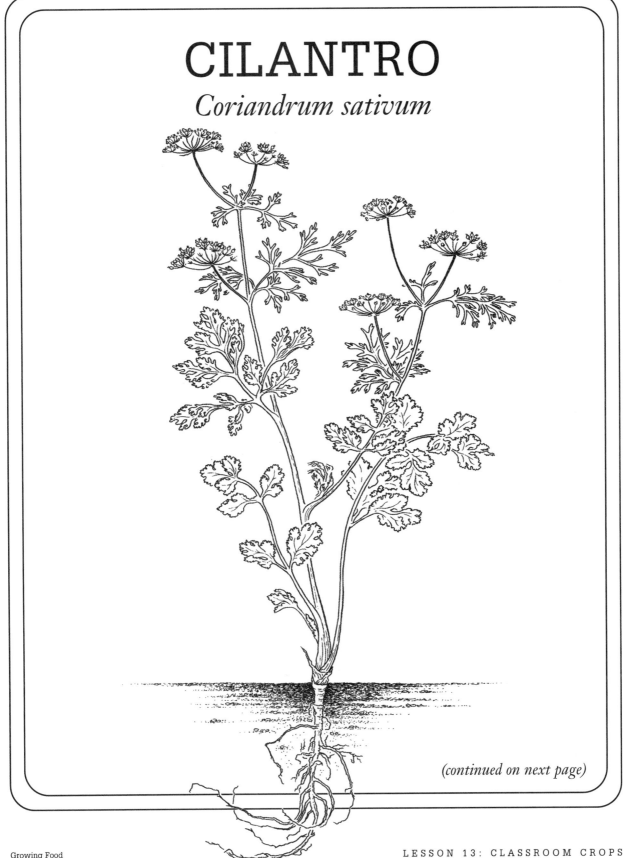

(continued on next page)

Name   Date

CILANTRO
Coriandrum sativum

ANNUAL HERB
The plant is called cilantro; its edible seeds are called coriander. Cilantro, also known as Chinese parsley, is a common ingredient in Asian cooking as well as in Mexican dishes. It is native to southern Europe and Asia Minor.

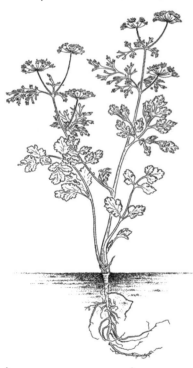

GROWING

Sow directly in full sun after danger of frost is past. For best results, plant in rows 12" apart. Thin plants to 6" apart when they are 2" tall. Easy to grow in any soil. Cilantro needs cool weather to grow well.

HARVESTING

For cilantro, pick leaves any time during the growing season before the plants flower. For coriander seeds, let the plants flower and go to seed. After the leaves and flowers have turned brown, the seeds are ready to harvest. Cut the plants, put them in a paper bag, and fasten with a tie. After a few weeks, turn upside down and shake the seeds off the plant into the bag.

COOKING

Chop fresh cilantro and use it in salsa. You also can use the leaves as a tangy garnish in salads, soups, and stir-fries. Use the seeds in meat and seafood dishes. Seeds also can be used to flavor breads, cookies, and cakes.

Start seeds in the Northeast	Days to germination	Planting depth	Plant spacing	Plant height	Preserve by
April–July	7–10	1/4"	6"	20"–28"	Drying

LESSON 13: CLASSROOM CROPS

Growing Food
©2007 Teachers College Columbia University

Name

Date

BECOMING FOOD SCIENTISTS : PLANTS : FOOD WEBS : AGRICULTURE : MAKING CHOICES

CUCUMBER

Cucumis sativus

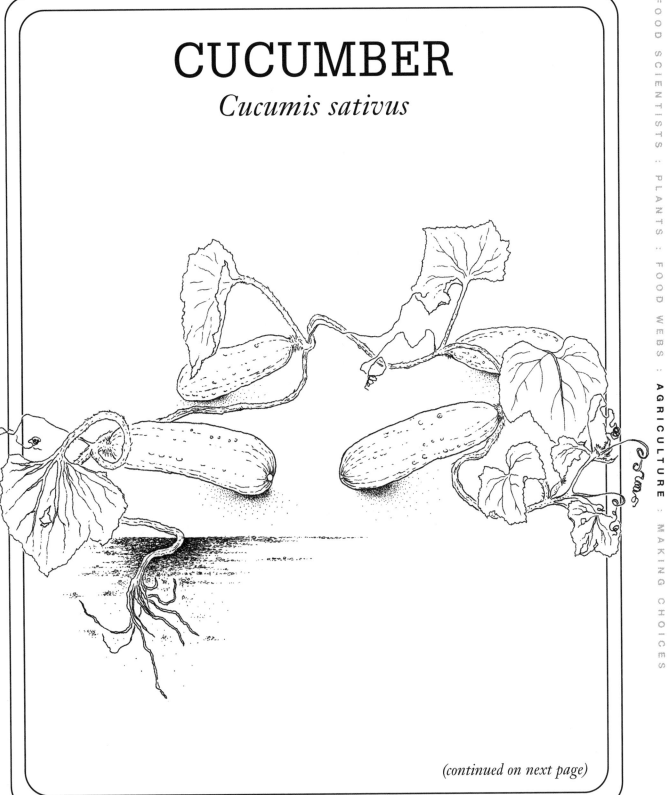

(continued on next page)

Name

Date

CUCUMBER
Cucumis sativus

ANNUAL VEGETABLE
Cucumbers grow fast and are easy to take care of. They thrive in the hot days of summer and can grow an amazing amount on a single hot day. One or two cucumber plants will give you a few cucumbers at a time all summer long.

GROWING

After all danger of frost and when the ground is warm, sow seeds 5" apart. Choose an area with full sun and well-drained soil. Thin plants to 20" apart when they are 2" tall. Cucumbers need lots of sunshine and water. Use an organic mulch, straw, hay, or leaves to control weeds. Cucumbers also grow well in patio containers — try 2 plants in an 18"-high, 18"-wide pot.

HARVESTING

Cucumbers are ready to pick once they are at least 5" long. Sometimes cucumbers hide under the leaves, so look carefully all over your plant to find them. Be sure to look at your plant every day, because the cucumbers grow very fast. If they get too big they will taste bitter.

COOKING

Use cucumbers fresh in salads or pickle them. Cucumbers are crispy and moist. They make a great snack right off the plant while you are gardening.

Start seeds in the Northeast	Days to germination	Days to harvest	Planting depth	Plant spacing	Preserve by
Late April–July	7–10	60	1/2"	20"	Pickling

Name   Date

DILL
Anethum graveolens

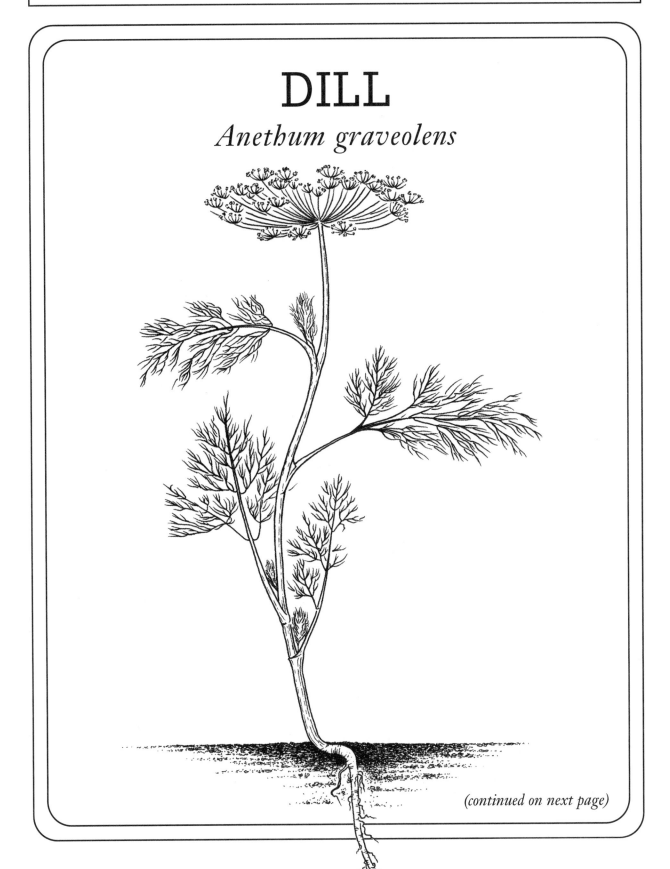

(continued on next page)

Name   Date

DILL
Anethum graveolens

ANNUAL HERB

Dill is an easy-to-grow herb. The seeds are used in making dill pickles. Fresh leaves are used to flavor salads, soups, meat, and fish. Dill is a native of southwest Asia but now is found all over Europe and North America.

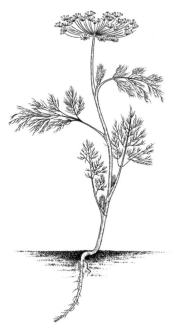

GROWING

Sow seeds directly in the garden in well-drained soil in a sunny location. Dill grows best in rows 9" apart. Thin plants to 9" apart when they are 2" tall. Dill is very easy to grow and needs a lot of room. Plant it in full sun for the best growth. Because of its size, plant dill with vegetables or in the back of an herb garden.

HARVESTING

Pick leaves anytime during the growing season. The youngest leaves are the tastiest. Harvest seeds when the flowers begin to turn brown. Put a paper bag over the seed heads and fasten the bag with a tie. After a few weeks, cut the stem off, turn upside down, and shake the seeds into the bag.

COOKING

Dill leaves are delicious in salads and soups. For pickling you can use fresh or dried seeds. Dill adds flavor to foods that may be somewhat bland, such as white fish or cucumbers. Slice cucumbers very thin, sprinkle them with salt, and let stand in a bowl for an hour or so. Pour off the liquid, and mix in a lot of chopped dill and a little sour cream.

Start seeds in the Northeast	Days to germination	Planting depth	Plant spacing	Plant height	Preserve by
April–July	7–14	1/4"	9"	26"–36"	Drying

Name   Date

ONION
Allium cepa

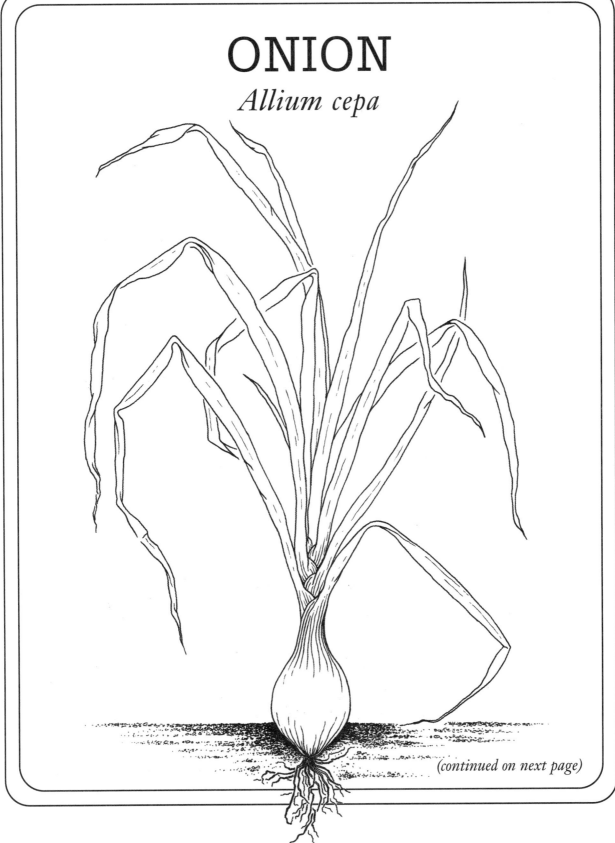

(continued on next page)

BECOMING FOOD SCIENTISTS : PLANTS : FOOD WEBS : **AGRICULTURE** : MAKING CHOICES

Name	Date

ONION
Allium cepa

ANNUAL VEGETABLE
Onions, garlic, chives, leeks, and shallots are related. They are members of the allium family. There are many different kinds of onions that vary in size and taste. Onions have a long growing season. If you plant onions directly from seed for your classroom crops, it is best to grow scallions or green onions.

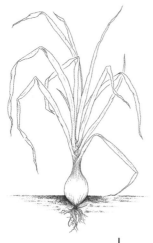

GROWING

Onions can be grown from seed, transplants, or onion sets. Start seeds indoors about 3 months before the last frost. Or sow seeds directly in the garden as soon as the soil can be worked in spring. Thin to 2" apart when plants are 3" tall. Plant onion sets or transplants after the last heavy frost. Push the sets into the soil so soil barely covers the bulbs. Space both the sets and transplants about 4" apart.

HARVESTING

When the onions are about the thickness of a pencil, they are ready to harvest as scallions. If you want small round onions, wait until the plants are about 1 month old. To harvest mature onions that you can store for a long time, wait until the plants are 3–4 months old and the tops are brown and lying on the ground.

COOKING

Onions add flavor to just about everything — from salsa to soup to sandwiches. When you thin the onions, you can use the young plants that you pull in place of chives.

Start seeds in the Northeast	Days to germination	Days to harvest	Planting depth	Plant spacing	Preserve by
Indoors: January/February Outdoors: after last frost	10–12	60	1/4"–1/2"	2"	Root cellar/cool storage

LESSON 13: CLASSROOM CROPS

Growing Food
©2007 Teachers College Columbia University

Name   Date

PARSLEY
Petroselinum crispum

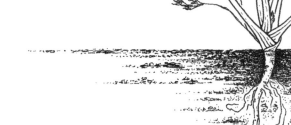

(continued on next page)

LESSON 13: CLASSROOM CROPS

177

Name   Date

PARSLEY
Petroselinum crispum

BIENNIAL HERB
Chewing parsley sweetens breath after eating onions or garlic. Parsley is native to Europe and western Asia. It is probably the best known of the culinary herbs.

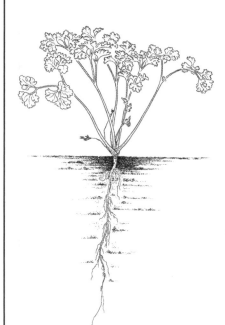

GROWING

Parsley seed usually is slow to germinate. Before planting, soak seeds in lukewarm water for an hour or more. For an early harvest, start seeds indoors. Or sow seeds outdoors in sun after the last frost. Thin or transplant seedlings when they are a few inches tall.

HARVESTING

Pick leaves any time after the plants are about 4" tall. For fresh use, pick early in the morning. The more you pick from the parsley plant, the bushier it will get.

COOKING

Use parsley leaves and stems fresh in stew, sauces, salads, and with vegetables and meats. This herb adds flavor to almost any dish. Chop some parsley leaves into very small pieces and add them to your favorite oil and vinegar salad dressing. You also can use parsley to make salsa verde.

Start seeds in the Northeast	Days to germination	Planting depth	Plant spacing	Plant height	Preserve by
April–June	21–28	1/4"	10"	12"–26"	Drying or freezing

BECOMING FOOD SCIENTISTS : PLANTS : FOOD WEBS : **AGRICULTURE** : MAKING CHOICES

PEPPER
Capsicum annuum

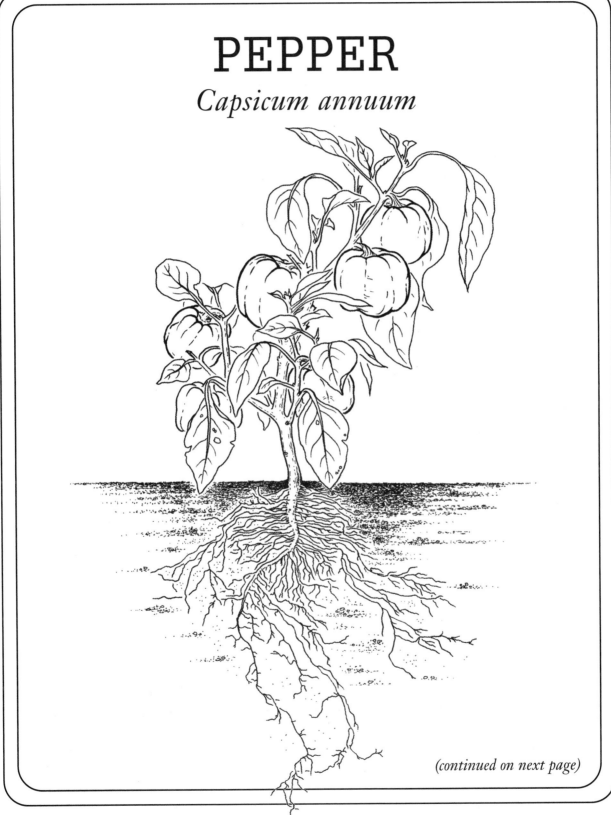

(continued on next page)

Name   Date

PEPPER
Capsicum annuum

ANNUAL VEGETABLE
Sweet pepper plants are medium-sized. They grow well even in a small garden. Peppers can be bell-shaped or long and thin. All peppers start out green and turn different colors as they mature and sweeten. Peppers can be red, yellow, orange, brown, cream, or even purple.

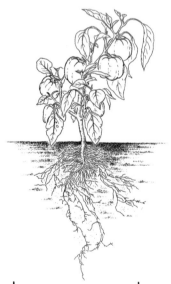

GROWING

Start seeds indoors 8 weeks before transplanting outdoors. Keep seeds moist in full sunlight. Or sow directly in the garden in a sunny location after danger of frost is over. Plant 2 seeds every 18". Thin to 1 plant every 18" when 3" tall. Add compost on top of soil when plants are 6" tall to increase production. If you also grow hot peppers, plant them in a separate area to avoid cross-pollination.

HARVESTING

You can pick peppers when they are any size. If you pick the peppers when small, that will help the plant produce more peppers. However, you may want to leave some on the plant to let them mature and sweeten and see what color they will become.

COOKING

Peppers are good raw and can be eaten any time as part of a meal or a snack. You can also sauté peppers with onions and garlic for a flavorful addition to stir-fries. Try chopping up peppers with tomatoes, onions, and cilantro for a great fresh salsa.

Start seeds in the Northeast	Days to germination	Days to harvest	Planting depth	Plant spacing	Preserve by
March–May	10–12	70–90	1/4"	18"	Drying or freezing

Name   Date

RADISH
Raphanus sativus

(continued on next page)

Growing Food
©2007 Teachers College Columbia University

LESSON 13: CLASSROOM CROPS

Name   Date

RADISH
Raphanus sativus

ANNUAL VEGETABLE
Radishes are most often thought of as round and red, but they can come in lots of shapes and colors. Pink, purple, and white are other common colors. Radishes can be shaped like olives or carrots.

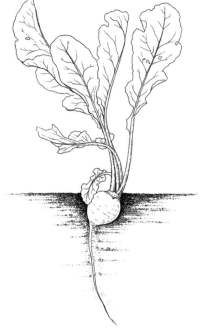

GROWING

Sow outdoors in full sun after all danger of frost. Cover seeds firmly with soil. When plants have 3–4 leaves, thin to 1" apart. For a continuous crop, sow every 10 days until warm weather arrives and again in fall until 30 days before frost. Radishes grow best in cool, moist soil. If radishes are grown in too much heat and with uneven watering, they will be bitter and tough.

HARVESTING

When plants look nice and bushy with lots of leaves, start checking under the soil to see how thick the radishes are. You can pick them when they are about an inch thick, or you can wait for them to get a little bigger. You will know the radishes are really ready to pick when they start peeking out from under the soil.

COOKING

Red radishes usually are eaten raw. Early spring radishes are crisp and tender. If you find them too hot and spicy, chop them into very small pieces and add them to salads. Radishes add color and flavor to vegetable trays. Try adding them to stir-fries.

Start seeds in the Northeast	Days to germination	Days to harvest	Planting depth	Plant spacing	Preserve by
May & August	4–7	28	1/2"	1"	Fresh use only

LESSON 13: CLASSROOM CROPS

Name　　　　　　　　　　　　　　　　Date

TOMATO
Lycopersicon lycopersicum

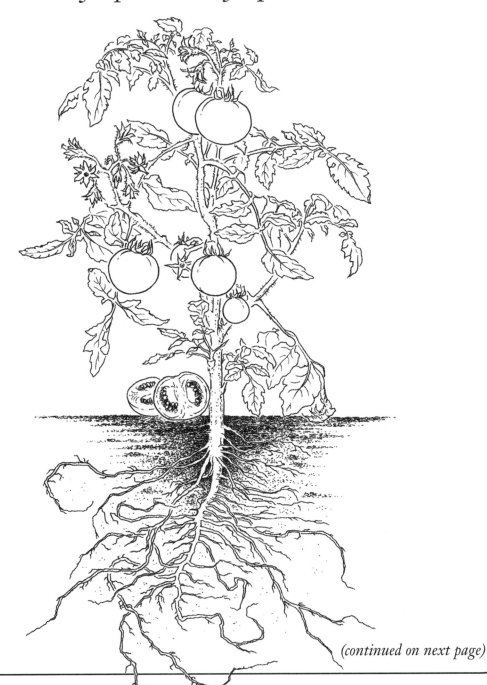

(continued on next page)

Name   Date

TOMATO
Lycopersicon lycopersicum

ANNUAL VEGETABLE
Homegrown tomatoes are delicious, and very different from most tomatoes we get in grocery stores. Although many tomatoes are red and round, some varieties can be yellow or even green when they are ripe. Tomatoes can have different shapes. Plum tomatoes are long and thin.

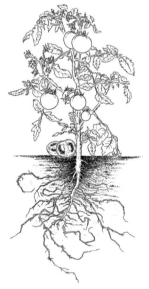

GROWING

Start seeds indoors in a sunny location 6 weeks before the last frost. Tomatoes cannot tolerate frost. Transplant outdoors in full sun when seedlings have 4–6 leaves and the weather is warm. Pick a very sunny spot in your garden; without sun you will get no tomatoes. Once tomatoes start to form and grow on your plant, you may need to stake the plants. This means pushing a thick stick or tomato cage into the soil and tying the plant to the stick or cage.

HARVESTING

The easiest way to test if tomatoes are ready to harvest is to try to gently pull them off the plant. When ripe, tomatoes will just about fall off in your hand.

COOKING

Tomatoes are delicious raw and can be eaten as a quick snack while you are gardening. They can be used in salads and salsas, or sliced and put on sandwiches. They can also be cooked into a sauce to put on pasta, or added to soups.

Start seeds in the Northeast	Days to germination	Days to harvest	Planting depth	Plant spacing	Preserve by
April	7–10	120	1/4"	24"	Canning or freezing

LESSON 13: CLASSROOM CROPS

Name   Date

Plant Information Table

THINGS TO CONSIDER WHEN PLANTING SEEDS				
Plant Name	Radish			
Days to Germination	4–7			
Days to Harvest	28			
Planting Depth	1/2"			
Plant Spacing	1"			
Plant Height				

Growing Food
©2007 Teachers College Columbia University

BECOMING FOOD SCIENTISTS : PLANTS : FOOD WEBS : **AGRICULTURE** : MAKING CHOICES

Investigating Soil

AIM

To investigate different kinds of soil.

SCIENTIFIC PROCESSES

- discover, investigate, compare

OBJECTIVES

Students will be able to:

- draw and describe some of the characteristics of soil;

- gain a new understanding of soil through hands-on soil investigations;

- discuss why farmers need to understand the characteristics of healthy soil.

OVERVIEW

This lesson furthers student understanding of soil and plant/soil interactions. Through hands-on investigations of local soil samples, students begin to gather data on the characteristics of healthy soil. Students compare two soil samples: one from a place where no plants are growing, the other from a place where plants are growing. By comparing their soil samples, students gather evidence that will help them begin to describe the characteristics of healthy soil. In the process, they discover that all soil is not alike. In their LiFE Logs, students reflect on what they have learned from their observations and about the terms farmers use to describe healthy soil. For homework, they study an illustration depicting a soil ecosystem and read about more of the indicators of healthy soil.

MATERIALS

For the teacher:
- *Soil Observations* experiment sheet
- *The Dirt on Soil* teacher note

For each group of 3–5 students:
- *Soil Observations* experiment sheet
- 1 cup soil from a place where plants are growing
- 1 cup soil from a place where no plants are growing
- 2 paper plates
- One sheet of chart paper
- Markers

For each student:
- *Healthy Soil* student reading
- *My Soil Observations* activity sheet
- (Optional) Hand lens and/or magnifying glass
- LiFE Log

PROCEDURE

Before You Begin:

- If you have not already done so, collect soil samples. You will need samples large enough to provide each group of students with at least one cup of each kind of soil. Be sure that one sample is sterile soil. Collect it from a place where nothing is growing. Make sure the other sample is fertile soil. Collect it from a place where plants are thriving.

- Follow the instructions on the experiment sheet for setting up the soil investigation and review the *My Soil Observations* activity sheet and *The Dirt on Soil* teacher note.

- Make copies of the *Healthy Soil* reading and the *My Soil Observations* activity sheet to distribute to each student. Make enough copies of the *Soil Observations* experiment sheet to distribute one copy to each group of students.

- Plan to save one cup of the fertile soil and one cup of the sterile soil from this lesson to use in Lesson 15.

- If you have not already done so, post the Module Question and the Unit 4 Question at the front of the class.

MODULE QUESTION

How does nature provide us with food?

UNIT QUESTION

How do we interact with nature to meet our food needs?

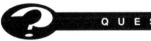
QUESTIONING

1. Review Module and Unit Questions

Review the Module and Unit questions with students. Explain that in this lesson the class is going to learn about what makes healthy soil and why farmers need to know about soil.

2. Think about Soil

Write the word "soil" on the board. Engage students in a discussion of the word to assess their current understanding. Encourage them to think about what they have already learned about soil through their seed-planting activity and what they have learned about decomposition. Record students' ideas on the board or on chart paper. If necessary, remind students that soil is essential for growing almost all terrestrial plants. They get nutrients from the soil. You may want to also point out that some free-floating aquatic plants, like duckweed, get their nutrients from the water. As you bring the discussion to a close, elicit students' ideas about this statement: "No soil, no life."

EXPERIMENTING

3. Investigate Soil Samples

Have the class work in small groups. Distribute one copy of the experiment sheet to each group and one copy of the activity sheet to each student. Introduce the soil investigation. In our small groups we will investigate two soil samples. Hold up the samples for all to see. This sample is labeled "Nothing Growing." This sample is labeled "Plants Growing." If the samples came from locations close to school, let students know where you collected them. Distribute the soil observation materials. You may wish to have student volunteers help you.

Have students follow along on the *Soil Observations* experiment sheet. Invite a student volunteer to read the questions out loud. Tell students to use these questions to guide their observations. Remind students to record their observations on the activity sheet as they examine the soil samples.

4. Display Observation Data

Once students have completed their observations, have them decide, within their small groups, which observations they wish to share with the whole class. Have them record those observations on the chart paper.

THEORIZING

5. Summarize and Reflect

Invite students to share their observations with the class. Have each group select a student representative to post the group's chart paper and share these observations with the class. Encourage other groups to ask questions and compare their findings.

APPLYING TO LIFE

6. LiFE Logs

Have students write the following in their LiFE Logs: "If I were a farmer, here's what I would hope to see in my soil." Have students write several sentences explaining what they would like to see in the soil and why. Remind them to cite evidence based on what they learned from their own soil observations.

SEARCHING

7. Distribute Homework

Give each student a copy of the *Healthy Soil* student reading. Have students complete the reading before you begin Lesson 15.

Remember to save one cup of each of the two different kinds of soil to use in Lesson 15.

Soil Observations

Students will make thorough observations of soil samples. They will use their senses to look at the soil, smell it, and feel it. Next, they will make quick sketches of what they observed.

Setup

1. Have students label the paper plates. They should label one plate "Plants Growing" and label the other plate "Nothing Growing."

2. Place 1 cup of fertile soil on the "Plants Growing" plate.

3. Place 1 cup of sterile soil on the "Nothing Growing" plate.

Procedure

1. Use the questions listed below to guide the soil observations.

2. Have students take turns examining the soil samples.

3. Have students record what they have seen. Make certain each student has a chance to be an observer and a recorder.

4. Have group members decide which observations they will record on the chart paper to share with the whole class.

Questions

1. *Do the two samples look the same? How are they alike? How are they different?* Use as many descriptive words as you can.

2. *Do you see any living creatures? Do you see anything that once was alive? Describe how it looks. What do you think it is? What kind of animals do you think live in soil?*

3. *What does each soil sample smell like? Do the samples smell the same or different?*

4. Touch each soil sample. *Do they feel the same or do they feel different?* Write at least one word to describe the texture of the soil.

5. Draw a quick sketch of what each soil sample looks like. If you have a magnifying glass or hand lens, use it to help you gather details for your sketch.

6. *What did you learn that you did not know before you made these observations?*

The Dirt on Soil

Soil is the layer of organic and mineral matter that covers much of the terrestrial land surface. Some scientists refer to it as "the skin of the earth." Although it varies in composition from place to place, in general it's made up of plant roots, plant and animal remains, air, water, rocks, and minerals. The process of making soil is a slow and continuous one. It includes the physical and chemical breakdown of rocks and the decaying of plant and animal remains. Soil is dynamic, constantly changing as the proportions of its components change.

Soils vary depending on the climate. Wind, water, and ice are constantly moving soil. The wind, for example, redistributes sandy soil by blowing it from one location to another. Water rushing down steep slopes often causes topsoil on the slopes to erode. Biological interactions cause soils to change as well. For example, burrowing animals, such as worms and moles, mix soils with their tunneling actions. Plant roots open channels in the soil, allowing water and air to enter. Fibrous plant roots near the soil surface, like grass roots, easily decompose and add organic matter to the soil.

In this lesson students are introduced to the basic components of soil. Based on their own observations, they begin to find out that there are different kinds of soil. In Lesson 15 students add to this knowledge by learning more about some of the characteristics of soil. They also add to their understanding of healthy soil. The term "healthy soil" has different meanings for different people. For farmers and gardeners, it refers to soil where plants can grow and thrive. Although soil is made up of mostly inorganic matter — sand, silt, and clay — it is the organic matter in the soil that is one of the key components of healthy soil. Organic matter, or humus, is a vital building block of soil. It helps soil retain water and nutrients. The amount of water soil holds depends on its components. For example, soil with a lot of sand in it does not hold water well. The water quickly passes through the coarse grains of sand. Soil with a lot of clay in it retains water and can become too wet for crops to thrive. Knowing how well soil holds water helps gardeners and farmers determine how often to water their plants.

Name   Date

Healthy Soil

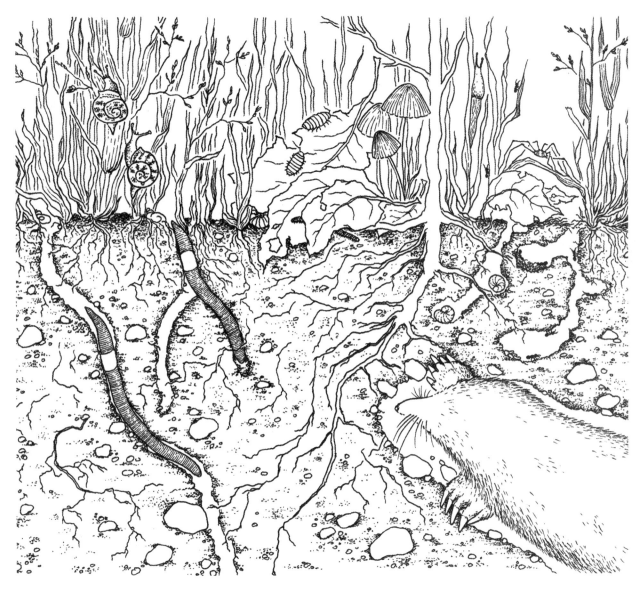

What is **healthy soil?** For a farmer, it means soil where crops grow well. How can you tell if soil is healthy? One sign is organic material. This indicates fertile soil where plants will thrive. Another sign of healthy soil is lots of plant and animal interactions. Look at the soil ecosystem on this page. Now find a soil food web. It begins with plants. Snails chomp on grass. Worms, sow bugs, ants, and bacteria feed on dead and decaying plants and animals, recycling nutrients into the soil. Moles burrow through the soil eating worms and insects. Their burrowing makes tunnels, which lets water and air into the soil. The organisms that live there need air and water to survive. All these interactions help make healthy soil and a place where more plants can grow.

| Name | Date |

My Soil Observations

OBSERVATIONS			
Soil Sample	See	Smell	Touch
Plants Growing			
Nothing Growing			

(continued on next page)

Name	Date

My Soil Observations

Plants Growing

Nothing Growing

LiFE Log

In your LiFE Log, write a few sentences describing what you learned from your soil observations.

Soil Texture

AIM

To understand some characteristics of healthy soil.

SCIENTIFIC PROCESSES

- **investigate, gather data, summarize**

OBJECTIVES

Students will be able to:

- **distinguish between different particles in two soil samples;**

- **analyze soil texture;**

- **describe differences between organic and sterile soil.**

OVERVIEW

In this lesson, students continue their investigation of soil. Through a reading, a simple activity, and a demonstration, students learn about soil structure. Soil includes three inorganic components — sand, silt, and clay — that vary in size and weight. Sand particles are the largest and heaviest. Clay particles are the smallest and lightest. Silt particles are in the middle. These particles also have different textures. Soil texture is the relative proportion of sand, clay, and silt that soil contains. To investigate soil texture, students rub some soil between their fingers. Sandy soil will feel gritty. Silt will feel silky or like flour. Clay soil will feel sticky. The soil-settling demonstration will help students see how the particles vary in weight. Allow at least two days for this activity so there is ample time for the soil particles to settle. These investigations help further students' understanding of the importance of soil to life. Without soil, there would be no plant life.

MATERIALS

For the teacher:
- *The Dirt on Soil* teacher note (p. 190)
- *Shake-n-Settle* experiment sheet
- 2 clear, 1-quart glass or plastic jars with secure lids
- Water (enough to fill the two jars)
- Spray bottle with water
- Soil samples from Lesson 14 (1 cup each of sterile soil and fertile soil)
- Two labels, one for each jar
- Chart paper
- Markers

For each group of 3–5 students:
- Small handful of soil
- Paper towel or paper plate

For each student:
- *Healthy Soil* student reading (p. 191)
- *Soil Particles* student reading
- *Shake-n-Settle Observations* activity sheet
- LiFE Log

PROCEDURE

Before You Begin:

- If you did not save the soil samples from Lesson 14, collect two soil samples. You will need one cup each of sterile soil and fertile soil for the demonstration and enough soil to give each group of students a small handful. Collect the soil from a place where nothing is growing and from a place where plants are thriving.

- Prepare labels for the two jars. Write "Nothing Growing" on one label. Write "Plants Growing" on the other.

- Review the **Shake-n-Settle** experiment sheet and follow the instructions for setting up the demonstration.

- You may wish to review the **The Dirt on Soil** teacher note.

- Make copies of the **Healthy Soil** and **Soil Particles** student readings and the **Shake-n-Settle Observations** activity sheet to distribute to students.

- If you have not already done so, post the Module Question and the Unit 4 Question at the front of the class.

MODULE QUESTION

How does nature provide us with food?

UNIT QUESTION

How do we interact with nature to meet our food needs?

 QUESTIONING

1. Review the Module and Unit Questions

Review the Module and Unit questions with students. Explain that in this lesson the class continues its study of soil by learning about soil structure and texture.

2. Discuss Soil Structure and Texture

Engage the class in a discussion of soil. *What are some facts you have learned about soil? Describe something about soil that you learned from your reading that you did for homework.* Compile a list of what students know about soil. *Now we're going to learn about soil structure and texture. How can we tell the texture of an object?* (Use our sense of touch.) *What are some words that describe different textures? During this activity you will be investigating soil texture and structure.*

 EXPERIMENTING

3. Investigate Soil Texture

Have students work in small groups. Invite student volunteers to help you distribute the student reading, paper towels or plates, and a handful of soil to each group of students. Give some groups a sample of the fertile soil and give the other groups a sample of the sterile soil. Have students record in their LiFE Logs which soil sample they are investigating.

Explain that you will spray the samples with water so the soil is damp. Then students will rub the soil between their fingers and think about its texture. Allow student groups several minutes to feel the soil and discuss within their small groups what they think the soil feels like. Have students record their descriptions of the soil texture in their LiFE Logs.

As a class, discuss soil texture. *Does the soil feel gritty? Does the soil feel slippery or silky to anyone? What other words would you use to describe the soil?*

SEARCHING

4. Learn about Sand, Silt, and Clay

Next, have students read *Soil Particles.* After they have finished, give them a few minutes to discuss what they learned within their groups. *Based on what you just read, do you think your group's soil sample has more sand, silt, or clay in it?* Make two columns on the board or on chart paper: "fertile soil" and "sterile soil." Accept all answers and record them on the chart. We'll compare your ideas now to the results of the Shake-n-Settle demonstration.

EXPERIMENTING

5. Begin the Demonstration

Introduce the soil demonstration. We will conduct a simple demonstration with our soil samples. (Hold up the samples for all to see.) These soil samples are labeled "Nothing Growing" and "Plants Growing."

Begin the demonstration. Follow the procedure outlined on the experiment sheet. *What do you predict will happen when we add water to these jars and shake them? Why do you think this will happen?* Accept all answers. Record them on the chart paper so students can look back at their ideas.

Have students take out their *Shake-n-Settle Observations* activity sheets. Invite two volunteers to add the water. Note the date and time and have students record it on the activity sheet. Make certain the lids are securely tightened. Shake the jars. Place the jars in a spot where the contents can settle without being disturbed. Ask for a student volunteer to keep track of the soil-and-water mix. Have that student record what time it is when the layers are formed. Record the date and time on the board so the class can record it on their activity sheets.

Note: You may wish to leave the jars overnight to allow ample time for the particles to settle

completely. If you do, be sure to leave a note next to the jars indicating that a science project is in progress so no one moves the jars.

6. Record Observations

Have students work in their small groups or in pairs to observe what has happened to the soil-and-water mix. If you use plastic jars, you can pass the jars around to each group. Be careful not to shake the jars once the soil has settled into layers. You may find it is easier to control this demonstration by keeping the jars level and in one spot. Have students take turns making their observations.

Help students see that the soil settles by the weight of the particles. The heaviest particles settle on the bottom; the lightest on the top.

THEORIZING

7. Build Theories about Soil

Ask students to think about what they have learned about soil. Encourage them to consider the role that soil plays in food production. Ask students to reflect on these questions: *What did you observe that was different about the soil where plants were growing that makes plants able to grow? What is your evidence?*

APPLYING TO LIFE

8. LiFE Logs

Have students take out their LiFE Logs and add to their Lesson 14 writing about soil, "If I were a farmer, here's what I would hope to see in my soil." Have students write several more sentences explaining what they would like to see in the soil and why. Remind them to cite evidence based on what they learned from their investigations of soil texture and structure.

Shake-n-Settle

Students investigate the inorganic and organic components of soil. Through their observations students discover that soil particles settle by weight and the organic matter floats at the top.

Setup

1. Label the two jars. Label one jar "Plants Growing." Label the other "Nothing Growing."

2. Fill the jar labeled "Plants Growing" about 1/3 full with fertile soil.

3. Fill the jar labeled "Nothing Growing" about 1/3 full with sterile soil.

Procedure

1. Show the students the jars partially filled with soil. In front of the class, fill each jar with water, put on the lid, and shake. Ask students to describe what they see and predict what they think will happen.

2. Use the questions below to guide students' observations. Remind students to record their answers on the activity sheet.

3. Have students observe how quickly the particles initially settle and note differences between the samples.

4. Put the jars in a safe location where they will not be disturbed.

5. Once the soil has settled, invite students to work in pairs or small groups to observe the two jars. Remind them to record their observations on their activity sheets.

6. After students have completed their observations, invite them to share their findings with the class.

Questions

1. Record the time that you begin shaking the jar. Record the time when most of the particles have settled. *How much time passed?*

2. *Do you notice any layers or separation?* Describe what you see.

3. Draw a sketch of how each sample settled in the jar. *Why do you think they settle this way? Hint:* Think about what would make things fall faster.

4. *What did you learn about the amount of sand, silt, and clay in each sample?*

Name   Date

Soil Particles

Soil contains different kinds of inorganic matter, including sand, clay, and silt. Soil is classified according to the proportion of sand, clay, and silt it contains. Particles of these three components are different sizes. The size of a particle affects how quickly water passes through the soil. For farmers, it's important to know a soil's characteristics because different kinds of plants grow well in different kinds of soil.

Clay

Particles of clay are too small to see with the naked eye. Small particles like clay do not let water pass through as easily as large particles do. Soils that retain water are not the best for growing crops and gardens. Clay soil is hard to manage. The soil gets too sticky when it's wet and too hard when it's dry.

Silt

Particles of silt are smaller than sand but larger than clay. Silty soils feel soft, almost silky. The space between silt particles is small, which means silt tends to hold water and nutrients better than sand. Silt is ideal for growing plants.

Sand

The largest particles in soil are sand particles, which you can see with the naked eye. When soil has a high percentage of sand particles, water and nutrients often drain too quickly due to the large size of the particles. Sandy soils are coarse and feel gritty. They need to be watered and fertilized often.

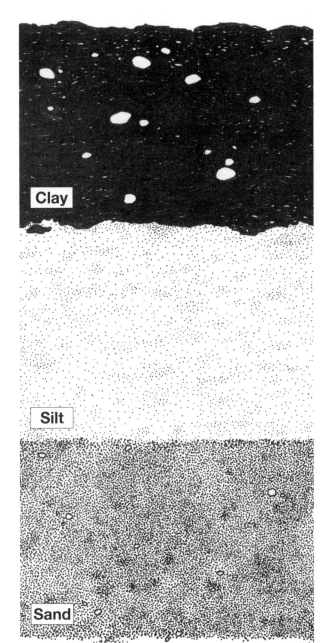

LESSON 15: SOIL TEXTURE   Growing Food
                                                        ©2007 Teachers College Columbia University

Name	Date

Shake-n-Settle Observations

OBSERVATIONS					
Soil Sample	Date	Start Time	Date	Stop Time	How Much Time Passed?
Plants Growing					
Nothing Growing					

Describe the layers:

_____

_____

_____

_____

_____

_____

LiFE Log

In your LiFE Log, sketch what you observed. Write a few sentences describing what you learned from your observations.

Crops and Weather

This lesson has two purposes. The first is to help students gain an understanding of the amount of knowledge that farmers need to have about climate and weather patterns in order to successfully farm their land. Without an understanding of climate, farmers wouldn't know what kinds of crops they could grow and they wouldn't know when they could plant their crops. The second purpose is to help students realize that farmers can't control the weather. In any given season the weather can help farmers have an abundant harvest or cause them to have no harvest at all. The student readings focus on three fictional tomato farmers and the challenges they faced during one growing season due to weather. These readings help students infer how weather can affect our food supply and the livelihood of farmers.

AIM

To infer how weather affects our food supply.

SCIENTIFIC PROCESSES

• **question, discover, explain**

OBJECTIVES

Students will be able to:

• **discuss what farmers need to know about weather patterns in their region;**

• **recognize why weather is important to farmers;**

• **generalize about the effect of weather and climate on our food supply.**

MATERIALS

For the teacher:
• *Weather, Climate and Growing Crops* sample conversation

For each student:
• *Changing Weather Conditions* student reading
• *Changing Weather Conditions Review* activity sheet
• LiFE Log

PROCEDURE

Before You Begin:

- Review the *Weather, Climate, and Growing Crops* sample conversation.

- Make copies of the *Changing Weather Conditions* student reading and *Changing Weather Conditions Review* activity sheet to distribute to students.

- If you have not already done so, post the Module Question and the Unit 4 Question at the front of the class.

MODULE QUESTION

How does nature provide us with food?

UNIT QUESTION

How do we interact with nature to meet our food needs?

 QUESTIONING

1. Review Module and Unit Questions

Review the Module and Unit questions with students. Explain that in this lesson they are going to learn why farmers need to know about the weather and climate where they grow crops.

2. Discuss How Weather Affects Farming

Encourage a whole-class discussion. *What if you were a farmer, what kinds of things would you need to know to be able to decide when to plant your crops? Do you think farmers can grow plants all year in all areas of the United States? Why do you think that? Do you think that it's different being a farmer in a state like North Dakota than in a state like Florida or Arizona? What makes you think that? How can we find out some answers to these questions?* See the *Weather, Climate, and Growing Crops* sample conversation for an example of how this conversation might go in your class.

 SEARCHING

3. Read Tomato Farming Stories

Distribute the student reading and activity sheet to students. Draw students' attention to the guiding questions at the beginning of the student reading. Invite student volunteers to read them out loud. Tell students to think about these questions as they read the stories. Have students silently read the stories about the three tomato farmers. When they have finished the reading, have them answer the review questions on the activity sheet.

 THEORIZING

4. Discuss the Effects of Weather and Climate

Ask a student volunteer to share her answer to the first question. *Does anyone else want to add anything? What evidence do you have to support your answer?* Invite students to discuss, as a class, whether or not they think all the farmers tried equally hard to have an abundant harvest. Remind them to cite their evidence to support their view. *Based on what you have learned, do you think that weather and climate can have an effect on what crops farmers grow and how much money they make? What makes you think this?*

 APPLYING TO LIFE

5. LiFE Logs

Write a paragraph that discusses how weather affects our food supply.

Weather, Climate, and Growing Crops

This sample conversation in the **Questioning** phase of the QuESTA cycle will help you guide your students though a conversation that will allow them to think deeply and thoughtfully about the topic they are about to study. During the conversation, students may ask questions, think about what they already know, speculate on answers to questions, and wonder about what they are going to learn. This is a guide. Feel free to adjust your questioning to the needs of your class.

MR. L: We have been learning about farming and what farmers need to know to be able to grow food for us to eat. Now we are going to learn about the effect of weather and climate on farming. *Can farmers grow plants all year in all areas of the United States?*

BETH: Plants can't grow all year where we live in New York. But last winter I visited my grandparents in Florida and they had plants growing in the winter.

FRANCISCO: My cousin is a farmer in Arizona and farms most of the year. It's much warmer where he lives.

MR. L: Right. In some states, people can farm most of the year. *Do you think it would be different to be a farmer in Minnesota compared to being a farmer in Florida?*

BETH: Sure. Minnesota gets really cold in winter and Florida doesn't. I know that farmers can grow oranges in Florida. But my grandfather told me that sometimes farmers in Florida worry when the weather gets cold. They are afraid it will hurt the orange crop. If you can't grow oranges when it's cold, I bet farmers can't grow oranges in Minnesota.

MR. L: That's good thinking. *Can you think of other ways that weather conditions like rain, or climate conditions like hot summers and warm winters can affect how plants grow?*

FRANCISCO: My cousin grows strawberries. He said that it rained a lot this spring and that was unusual. Most of the time the spring is warm and sunny. He said his strawberries don't have much flavor because there weren't enough sunny days. Some of the berries were rotten in the fields, too.

MR. L: Interesting. *If the weather affects the farmer's crops, do you think this will have an impact on how much money he makes?*

FRANCISCO: My cousin said he didn't have as many strawberries to take to the market to sell because of all the rain. He's not going to have as much money as in other years.

MR. L: That's an important observation. Weather and climate can have an effect on how much money a farmer can make. Now let's read about some tomato farmers and how weather and climate affected their crops.

Name   Date

Changing Weather Conditions

Guiding Questions

- *What have you learned about the difference between climate and weather?*
- *Why is it important for farmers to understand climate and weather?*
- *Why do you think weather conditions affect crops?*
- *What evidence do you have to support your conclusions?*

Here are stories about three tomato farmers who live in Kansas. The farms are located in different parts of the state. Each farmer grows three acres of tomatoes. All three farmers know a lot about growing tomatoes. They work hard to have healthy growing conditions. The farmers want to produce high-quality, tasty tomatoes that they can sell.

Last year the farmers had very different experiences growing their tomatoes. Part of this was due to the weather conditions where they farm in Kansas. In each story you will learn about the weather conditions and how they affected the tomato crop. You will discover how important it is for farmers to understand about the weather, climate, and growing conditions where they farm.

Climate information tells farmers how the weather has acted over many years. They can find out the rainiest month or the last day of freezing temperatures. For example, the climate in Kansas is good for growing tomatoes. The weather is what is happening now. For example, a change in the weather could cause a sudden drop in temperature. Or there could be a heat wave. Looking at climate information, farmers know there are cold winters and hot summers in Kansas. They can predict lots of sun, warm summers, and rain during the tomato-growing season. It's harder to predict the weather conditions. Kansas is famous for tornadoes and violent thunderstorms. Farmers can't predict these sudden weather changes when they do their planning for the growing season. In each story, you'll discover how each farmer was affected by changing weather conditions.

Bill Tucker's Farm

Farmer Tucker lives in the southern part of Kansas. Based on climate information for his area, he knew when he could plan to plant his tomatoes outside. He started his tomato seeds inside his greenhouse in March, when it was still very cold outside. This helped the plants get off to a good start. By the end of April it had warmed up enough so that Farmer Tucker could move the plants outside. May was a good growing month. It was

(continued on next page)

Name   Date

Changing Weather Conditions

sunny and warm most of the time. These conditions helped the tomato plants grow tall and strong. However, in June there was a big hailstorm. The hail knocked off many of the flowers. Without the flowers, there would be no tomatoes. The storm also brought high winds. The winds blew over the plants and weakened their stems and root systems.

Farmer Tucker had not planned for this storm. It took almost two weeks for the plants to begin to recover, and Farmer Tucker realized they would never fully recover. July and August were hot and sunny. Farmer Tucker made sure the tomato plants had enough water. The weather conditions in July and August were perfect for growing large, healthy tomatoes. However, Farmer Tucker's tomato production was low. It was much lower than he had planned. He only had about 20 tomatoes on each plant. In spite of the fact that most of the summer had wonderful weather conditions for growing, that one hailstorm in June had had a strong impact on his harvest. Farmer Tucker was very worried about how his family would make ends meet. Because of the storm, he and his family would only make about half the money they usually did. One change in the weather changed his income.

Carla Fernandez's Farm

Farmer Fernandez lives in the central part of Kansas. Using what she knows about the climate in Kansas, she planned when to plant her tomato crop. Sometimes there is not enough rain for her plants to grow. Farmer Fernandez has irrigation ditches in case she needs to give the plants water. In March, when it was still cold outside, she planted her tomato seeds in her greenhouse to get her plants off to a good start. It stayed cold throughout April in her part of Kansas, so she waited until May to move the plants outside. May was a warm month. Luckily, there was plenty of rain in May for her plants and to fill the ditches in case the weather turned dry.

Without extra help from Farmer Fernandez, the tomato plants grew healthy and strong. There was good growing weather throughout June, July, and August. It was hot and dry. Because of the May rain, Farmer Fernandez was able to give her tomato plants plenty of water every day from her irrigation ditch. By the middle of August, her tomatoes were ready. She had a record crop of about 40 tomatoes per plant! This was more than she had planned, which meant she would have more tomatoes to sell. She was excited that she would earn more money for this year's crop of tomatoes. She decided to plan a long vacation to a warm island where she could relax after the long farming season.

(continued on next page)

Name	Date

Changing Weather Conditions

Sandy Marshal's Farm

Farmer Marshal lives in northern Kansas. Due to the climate in her part of Kansas, she knows that she can't plant tomatoes outside until early May. She planned ahead and planted her seeds in the greenhouse so they would be ready by May. The weather conditions in early May were just right for moving the tomato plants outside. It was warm and there was plenty of rain. Farmer Marshal thought her plants would grow just fine. But the weather in June was unusual. It was a cold, gray, rainy month. Although the plants grew, there were very few flowers.

Farmer Marshal knew the tomatoes needed plenty of bright sunlight to grow enough to make flowers. Without flowers, there would be no tomatoes. Farmer Marshal began to get worried. She hoped the weather would be what she expected in Kansas in July. However, July and August brought more gray, rainy days. The weather report said it was the coolest, rainiest summer on record since 1897! Farmer Marshal's plants produced some tomatoes, but without a lot of sun, most of the tomatoes stayed green. Very few got ripe and turned red. On top of everything else, all of the rain caused many of the tomatoes to become moldy while they were still on the plant. Farmer Marshal had a very poor harvest. She only had about eight tomatoes from each plant. Without tomatoes to sell, she had no money. She did not know how she was going to pay her mortgage and the rest of her bills. After the season was over, she decided her only choice was to go to the bank to ask for a loan.

Name

Date

Changing Weather Conditions Review

Answer the following questions.

1. Write a few sentences to describe the effect the weather had on the tomato growing season on each farm.

_____

_____

_____

_____

_____

_____

_____

2. Do you think all the farmers tried equally hard to have a good harvest? Why or why not?

_____

_____

_____

_____

(continued on next page)

Name	Date

Changing Weather Conditions Review

3. What would it be like to have a job that is so affected by the weather?

_____

_____

_____

_____

4. Imagine you are going to interview one of these farmers. Think about three questions you would like to ask the farmer about his or her experiences last season. Write your questions in this space. Which farmer would you interview? Why would you choose this farmer?

_____

_____

_____

_____

_____

_____

_____

_____

_____

(continued on next page)

BECOMING FOOD SCIENTISTS : PLANTS : FOOD WEBS : **AGRICULTURE** : MAKING CHOICES

Name   Date

Changing Weather Conditions Review

5. Next time you are in the grocery store and you see tomatoes, will you wonder about the farm where they were grown? Why or why not?

_____

_____

_____

_____

_____

_____

BECOMING FOOD SCIENTISTS : PLANTS : FOOD WEBS : **AGRICULTURE** : MAKING CHOICES

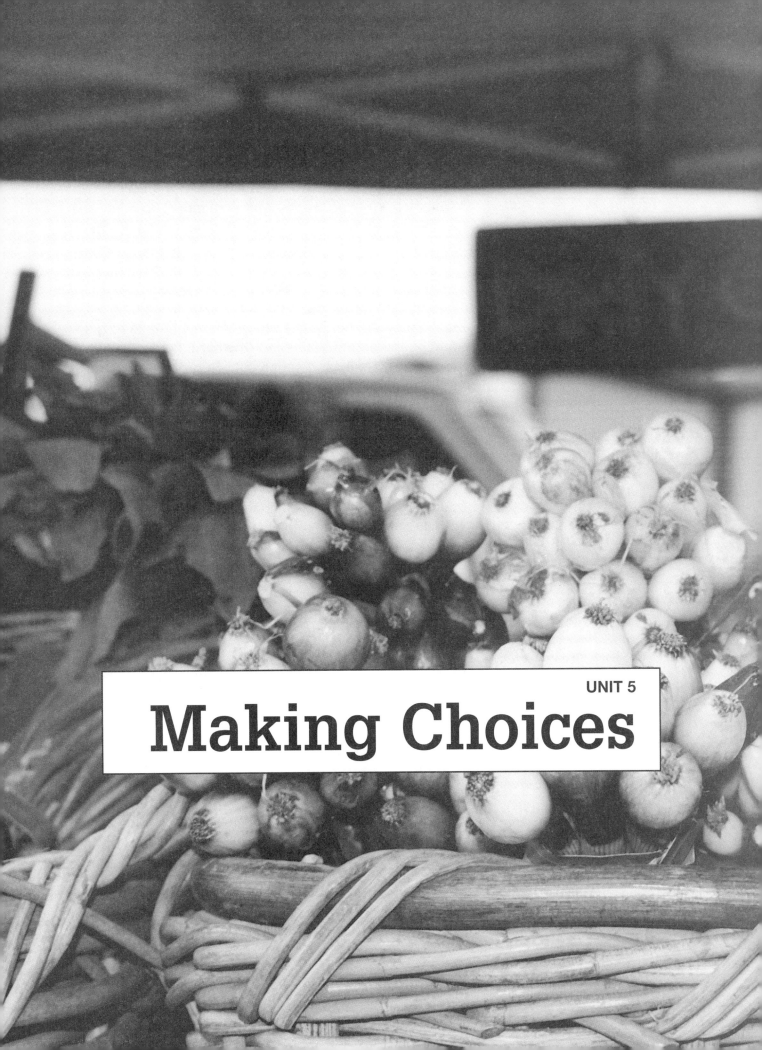

UNIT 5

Making Choices

Regional Eating

AIM

To use regional eating maps to research what it means to eat locally and seasonally.

SCIENTIFIC PROCESSES

• question, search, theorize, apply

OBJECTIVES

Students will be able to:

• identify their region, locate their state on a map, and learn what foods are available from local farmers in their regions in the different seasons;

• understand what it means to eat locally/regionally and seasonally in general and in particular within their own region/state;

• apply the seasonal-foods information for a particular region in designing seasonal menus.

OVERVIEW

Thus far, students have been exploring the Unit 4 Question, *How do we interact with nature to meet our food needs?* In investigating this question, students examined the world of agriculture and the role humans play in producing the foods we eat. This lesson focuses on understanding our roles as active consumers and community members in our local food system. In this lesson, students use the regional eating maps to gain a conceptual understanding of what it means to eat locally/regionally and seasonally. In groups, students learn what fruits and vegetables are available by season in a particular region and design seasonal menus. Groups present their results to the class and discuss similarities, differences, and new questions that arise. The class also discusses the benefits of eating locally and explores ways in which students will, for homework, take action to incorporate local foods into their individual, family, and community diets.

MATERIALS

For the teacher:
• *The Benefits of Eating Local Food* lesson resource
• *Taking Action* lesson resource
• *Think Globally, Eat Locally* teacher note

For the class:
• Fruits and/or vegetables (or pictures of them) corresponding to each region for the current season
• Wall map of the United States
• 8 (or more) sheets of chart paper & markers
• A few thumbtacks

• (Optional) Fruits and/or vegetables from farmer's market or other local sources. If possible, bring foods you think the students might not be familiar with.

For each student:
• *Eating Locally and Seasonally* student reading
• *Regions 1–8* student readings
• *Bringing It Home* activity sheet
• LiFE Log

PROCEDURE

Before You Begin:

- Gather materials.

- Review *The Benefits of Eating Local Food* and *Taking Action* lesson resources, and the *Think Globally, Eat Locally* teacher note.

- (Optional) If you brought in food, prepare it for tasting, i.e., by washing, cutting, displaying, etc.

- Make copies of the *Regions 1–8* and *Eating Locally and Seasonally* student readings and the *Bringing It Home* activity sheet for each student.

- If you have not already done so, post the Module Question and the Unit 5 Question at the front of the class.

MODULE QUESTION

How does nature provide us with food?

UNIT QUESTION

How can we use the science we've learned to make food and agriculture choices?

 QUESTIONING

1. Introduce Unit 5 Question

Review with students the Module Question and the first four Unit questions.

Discuss what we have learned about interactions in nature and how humans interact with and alter nature's systems to provide for our own food needs. Then, introduce the Unit 5 Question and explain that we are going to learn about our roles as consumers and community members in our local food system.

2. Consider Food Miles

Pose the following questions for discussion. These questions can be discussed in pairs (students interviewing each other and reporting back), small groups, and then as a class, or written in students' LiFE Logs and then discussed. By now students are more aware of how food is grown, harvested, processed, and so forth from the previous lessons in this module, so challenge them to describe these processes for some of their favorite foods. *Think about the last thing you ate. Do you know where it came from? Who grew and harvested it? How many miles did it travel to get to you? Can you trace one food item all the way back to its origins? Can you say how and where it grew or was formed and how it was harvested, processed, transported, packaged, and made available to you?*

3. Discuss Eating Locally

Discuss the idea of eating within your local food system. Depending on the above discussion, the following questions can guide you. *Does anyone have an idea of what it means to eat locally? Has anyone ever heard about eating locally grown food? What do you think it means if a food was grown locally? Has anyone ever eaten something locally grown? How did you know?*

Discuss what "local" means. Refer to the lesson resource *The Benefits of Eating Local Food* to guide this discussion. Return to this definition at the end of the class and ask students to come up with their own definition after they work with the regional maps and seasonal foods.

Talk to your students about how an important part of eating locally is eating with the seasons. As an example, use eating tomatoes during the summer and early fall months when they are available and then not again until the next year. *Can anyone tell me what it means to eat seasonally?* Talk about the benefits of eating seasonally.

Discuss the reasons that many people are moving toward eating within their local food system.

Today we're going to find out what's in season in our region so we can start eating locally and seasonally!

 SEARCHING

4. Learning about Climatic Regions

Distribute *Eating Locally and Seasonally*. Have students refer to the map showing all eight regions. *Does anyone have an idea of how we get eight different regions on this map? Why do you think it was divided this way?*

Talk about how the U.S. was divided by climatic region because of how much climate affects what farmers can grow and when crops can be harvested. Try to reinforce what students learned about climate and weather in Lesson 16.

Distribute the regional eating maps. Have students find their region and pull out the map of their region with the corresponding seasonal foods. They should also look over the other regional maps to get an idea of the foods grown in different parts of the country.

Quickly discuss the fact that each of these regions has many local food systems within it. *Look at the maps. Can you figure out what other states might qualify as local for our community?* Not all the states in your region are close enough to be considered local.

Remind students that these are climate-region maps and some regions are large; therefore, eating locally means a much smaller scale (return to definitions if necessary). Students can think about the seasonal boundaries as the outermost boundaries of sustainability. Ideally, they would draw from their own local food system first (maybe somewhere between 100 and 300 miles), and then expand into their regional seasonal food system. Reinforce the idea that the fewer miles your food travels the better.

5. Using Regional Food Guides

The regions are helpful for knowing what foods are available at what times of year. Once students have found their regions, have them identify their state within their region and then their city with a star. Have students read what foods are available and in what season. Engage students in a discussion of what they have read. *Were you surprised by what you read? Are there any foods that you recognize and eat often? Is there any food that isn't familiar?* As homework, select volunteers to find information about foods that are not familiar to students and report back to the class.

What foods do you eat when they are not in season in your region? How do you get them? Now that you can see what's available to you in different seasons and to people living in other regions, what are some benefits to eating locally? What are some drawbacks?

Talk about how eating locally allows consumers to answer many of the questions students were trying to answer about their favorite foods, like where they were grown and harvested and how many miles they traveled before they got to them.

(The following are optional, depending on if you have brought local foods in for the students to try.) Present the foods you brought in. Talk about the foods from local sources. Have students taste the foods.

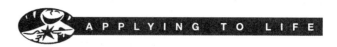 **APPLYING TO LIFE**

6. Planning Seasonal Meals

Divide students into eight groups. Assign each group one region to study. In these groups students will design seasonal menus for their assigned region. Have them create at least one meal for each season using the foods listed on their maps. Students can write or draw their menus on large sheets of chart paper. Have the groups elect one or two people to present their work to the class.

Facilitate a discussion about the differences and similarities between seasonal meals of different regions. Have any new questions come up for the students? Ask students to think about and discuss how their lives would be different if they ate only or mostly local food instead of global food.

7. Visualizing Food Miles

Present the foods or pictures of foods you brought that correspond to each region for whatever season you are in. (For example, if it's winter you could bring an orange for Region 6, a potato for Region 1, etc. Some foods may correspond to multiple regions depending on the season.)

Have students match the foods to the appropriate regions as you present them. Place a thumbtack on your large U.S. map corresponding to the town where your school is located.

For each food item elect a volunteer to put a thumbtack on a state within the region that the food corresponds to. Have another student measure the distance between the thumbtacks using a meter stick and have each student individually convert the centimeters (or inches) to miles using the scale on the map. Students should get an idea of how far many foods typically travel. Discuss.

8. Develop Strategies for Action

Using the lesson resource *Taking Action*, discuss with students possible ways to start eating locally in their communities.

Other activities your class could do together include writing a class cookbook with different meals for each season or taking a challenge to eat local foods for a specific length of time — you and your students can decide what length of time is appropriate. Depending on the season this will be more or less difficult, so discuss that with students. Maybe eating 25 percent

local food for a week is possible. Perhaps you eat something local at each meal for a week or a month.

9. Homework

Discuss the *Bringing It Home* activity sheet with your students. Review the questions at the beginning (all students should answer these questions) and discuss the options for the second part of the sheet.

There are several choices for the second part of this assignment; students will each do two, but some might want to do more.

The Benefits of Eating Local Food

There are many reasons to buy local food. You and your students may come up with additions to this list. Local food systems are economically sound, ecologically sustainable, and socially just.

It Tastes Better

Food that travels long distances is picked before it's fully ripe and some is treated with chemicals to prevent natural decomposition processes. Food that ripens in a refrigerated truck doesn't taste very good. Just think about that peach you bought in March. Food grown in your community is probably picked within 48 hours of the time you buy it.

It's Better for You

Studies show that produce loses nutrients quickly, so the sooner it's eaten after harvest, the better. Even produce that was frozen or canned just after harvest may be better than produce that has spent a week in a refrigerated truck.

You're Supporting Family Farms

Today less than two percent of our population is made up of farmers. In general farmers get less than ten cents of every dollar we spend on food due to the costs of processing, transportation, and distribution. Local farmers who sell directly to consumers through farmer's markets and Community Supported Agriculture programs (CSAs) avoid these costs and get to keep more of what we pay them.

You're Building Community

You create a sense of community when you cultivate and maintain relationships with farmers and other consumers, and community members.

You're Preserving Open Space

This is especially true where farmland surrounds urban areas, as in New York and California, where farmland is much more profitable when developed than when it's used to grow food. Buying locally grown foods shows that we value farmland as undeveloped, open space for all to enjoy. It also shows that farmland can be profitable.

Family Farms Are Environmentally Sustainable

Buying locally means reducing transportation costs, therefore relying less on fossil fuels. Meals made from imported ingredients can account for four times the energy and greenhouse gas emissions of equivalent meals made with locally grown ingredients.

Buying from family farmers supports their efforts to preserve soils and prevent erosion. Unlike most huge farming operations, family farmers often rotate crops, use cover crops and ecologically sound practices for managing pests, and, particularly for animals, handle wastes more efficiently.

Eating Locally Is Good for the Future

Supporting your local farmer ensures there will be farms tomorrow. Remember, "no farmers, no food."

Taking Action

Discuss with students actions that you can take. Here are some suggestions to guide your discussions.

Learn Your Region's Seasonal Foods

Learn what foods are in season in your area (using the maps in this lesson) and try to build meals around these foods. Everything you eat does not have to be local, and in fact it will be very difficult to eat all local foods, but try to incorporate many of the foods you learn about.

Shop Your Local Farmer's Market

To find the farmer's markets in your area visit *www.ams.usda.gov/farmersmarkets/map.htm*, where they are listed by state. Another way to get local produce is to join your local Community Supported Agriculture program. With Community Supported Agriculture (CSA), you basically invest in the farm by supporting the farmer at the beginning of the season and reaping rewards throughout the year.

Eat Local Foods When You Eat Out

Talk to the manager or chef at your favorite local restaurant. Find out if any of the food served is local and if it's possible to increase the number of local foods served.

Host a Harvest Party

Throw a party in your home, classroom, school, or community that features locally grown, seasonal foods.

Make a Directory

Create a directory of local food sources for your community that lists farmers' markets, CSAs, and restaurants that emphasize local foods, farm stands, urban farms, community gardens, food co-ops, local bakeries, meat processors, etc.

Put Food Away

Buy extra amounts of your favorite foods, like strawberries and tomatoes, when they are in season and experiment with preservation methods like canning, freezing, and drying that will allow you to enjoy them year-round.

Start a Garden

Plant a garden, a few pots, or window boxes and try growing some of your own food. There are varieties of tomatoes that grow well in pots and herbs are great in window boxes. Consider joining a community garden.

Think Globally, Eat Locally

"Think globally, eat locally." What does this expression mean? Right now most of the food Americans eat travels an average of 1,500 miles from the farm to our plates. Currently it is possible to go to the supermarket and find almost any food from anywhere at any time. This can be great for us as consumers because it means we feel we have lots of choices about what to eat whether it's July or January. Back when most people still grew their own food, they ate what was in season or what they had preserved, and that was it. For most people that meant no fresh tomatoes or strawberries in the winter. It also meant that if a freeze or a flood ruined your potatoes you'd have to figure out something else to eat all winter. Today, however, if the orange crop in Florida is ruined we can get oranges from California or Spain, even if we live in Chicago. Having what is called a global food system also means that for those of us who don't live in tropical climates we can eat bananas and mangoes anytime we want to. While many of us like all the choices that a global food system provides us, there are others of us who are worried about the impact of our current system on the environment, local economies, communities, farmers, and consumers, not to mention how food tastes.

Why is there concern about our current food system? Thanks to advances in technology that allow food to keep in storage longer for less money, food today travels farther and is controlled by a smaller number of global corporations than ever before. All this means that people are becoming further and further removed from their food sources both by distance and by processing. Instead of feeling as if we have endless choices we are losing power over what we eat and where it comes from. Most of us have no idea how, where, or by whom our food is grown, produced, processed, and shipped. There is, however, an alternative — one that's good for communities, farmers, the environment, and our taste buds: a regional, local, sustainable food system. Eating locally gives you a voice in your community about how land gets used, what pollutants end up in your local waters and soils, and the physiological and financial health of the community. It reminds us that, as the poet-farmer Wendell Berry has said, "eating is an agricultural act."

Eating locally also means adjusting our choices, appetites, and eating patterns to Nature and her seasons — enjoying fruits and vegetables at their peak and experimenting with new vegetables when familiar ones are out of season. Summer becomes an opportunity to freeze, can, or dry favorite fruits and vegetables while they're plentiful and delicious. Winter is a great time to combine canned, frozen, dried, and stored produce with local meats and dairy products that are available year-round. Furthermore, not *everything* you eat has to be local. For most of us that would be impossible and impractical. Produce is ideal food to buy locally because its weight and perishability make transportation across long distances wasteful. And because local tomatoes and peaches taste so much better than "jetlagged" ones! Check out the lesson resources to find out more about why eating locally is so important and what you, your students, and your community can do to get started.

Name   Date

Eating Locally and Seasonally

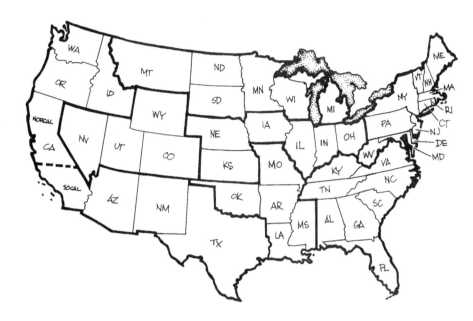

"Think globally, eat locally." Right now, most of the food we eat travels an average of 1,500 miles from the farm to our plates. That's halfway across the country! When you go into a super-market you can buy anything you want, whenever you want it. You wouldn't even know there were seasons! But what if we ate mostly what was in season and grown in our local region? Many people think eating locally and seasonally is a good idea because it's better for communities, farmers, the environment, and our taste buds. Eating locally means adjusting our diets to nature and the seasons. It means enjoying fruits and vegetables at their peak and experimenting with new vegetables when familiar ones are out of season. Many foods grow in different places and at different times for various reasons, primarily differences in regional climates.

On this map, the United States is divided into eight regions based on climate. You might already know that the southern part of the United States has milder weather than the northern part, so different foods grow in those regions at different times of the year. This means people in Florida eat a very different seasonal diet than people living in Montana. Where do you live? First find your region on the map above. Then find the map on the following pages that highlights only your region. This regional map lists the fruits and vegetables that are in season during the winter, spring, summer, and fall. Check out the foods that are listed and think about how your life would be if you ate a seasonal diet. In addition to the fruits and vegetables listed on these pages, there are many other foods available during each season in your region. You may want to go to farmers' markets, visit farms, or search in books or on the Internet to add to the list of what is available in each season. Creating a more complete list will give you a better idea about what it would be like to eat seasonally in your region.

Name   Date

Region 1

ME, VT, NH, MA, CT, RI, NY, PA, NJ, DE, MD, WV

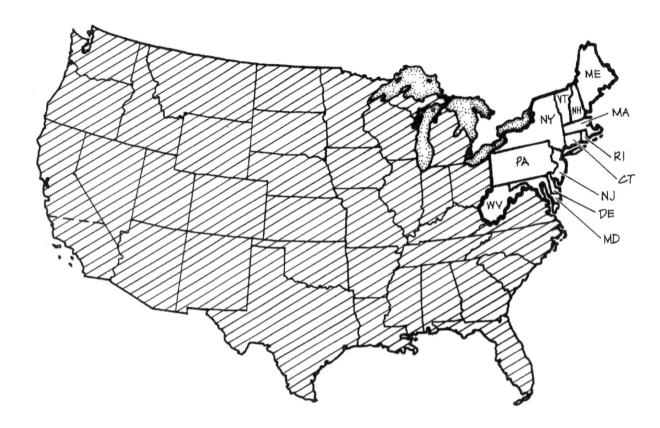

WINTER	SPRING	SUMMER	FALL
Apples CS	Asparagus	Arugula	Apples
Beets CS	Cauliflower	Blueberries	Brussels sprouts
Carrots CS	Fiddleheads	Corn	Fennel
Jerusalem artichokes	Lettuce	Cucumbers	Garlic
Parsnips CS	Peas	Eggplant	Mushrooms
Potatoes CS	Radishes	Green beans	Pears
Rutabagas CS	Rhubarb	Peaches	Squash (Summer, Winter)
Sweet potatoes CS	Spinach	Tomatoes	Turnips

CS (cold storage): These are stored after harvest for use in multiple seasons.

LESSON 17: REGIONAL EATING

Name   Date

Region 2

MT, ND, SD, MN, WI, MI

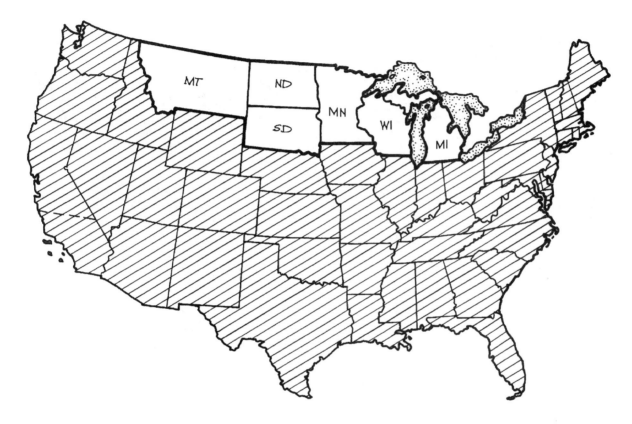

WINTER	SPRING	SUMMER	FALL
Apples CS	Asparagus	Carrots	Apples
Beets CS	Green onions	Cucumbers	Beets
Cabbage CS	Greens	Eggplant	Broccoli
Carrots CS	Mushrooms	Green beans	Cauliflower
Kohlrabi CS	Potatoes CS	Raspberries	Daikon
Onions CS	Radishes	Squash (Summer)	Fennel
Parsnips CS	Raspberries	Strawberries	Melons (late)
Potatoes CS	Spinach	Tomatoes	Squash (Winter)

CS (cold storage): These are stored after harvest for use in multiple seasons.

Name   Date

Region 3

ID, WA, OR, CA (northern)

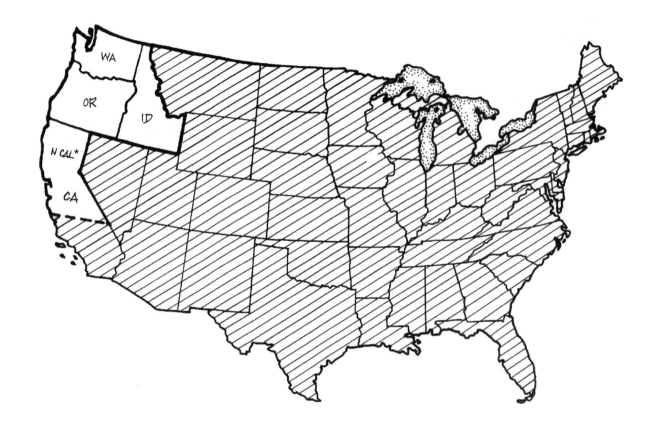

WINTER	SPRING	SUMMER	FALL
Arugula	Beets	Corn	Artichokes
Broccoli	Carrots	Cucumbers	Cabbage
Cabbage	Cauliflower	Green beans	Carrots
Citrus	Greens	Melons	Lettuce
Kiwis	Lettuce	Mushrooms	Persimmons
Leeks	Onions	Peppers (Hot,	Rutabagas
Potatoes	Peas	Sweet)	Squash (Summer)
Squash (Winter)	Rhubarb	Strawberries	Tomatoes
		Tomatoes	

*Changes in climate, even within regions, may result in changes in seasonal availability or harvest times of some foods.

LESSON 17: REGIONAL EATING

Growing Food
©2007 Teachers College Columbia University

BECOMING FOOD SCIENTISTS : PLANTS : FOOD WEBS : AGRICULTURE : MAKING CHOICES

Name   Date

Region 4

VA, NC, SC, GA, FL, KY, TN, AL

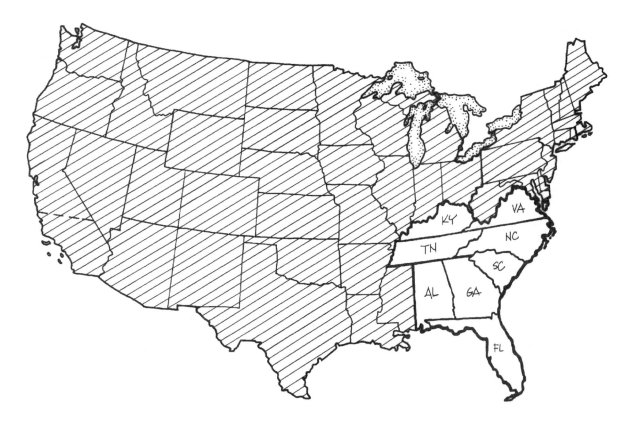

WINTER	SPRING	SUMMER	FALL
Apples	Blueberries	Brussels sprouts	Bell peppers
Avocados	Broccoli	Cantaloupes	Broccoli
Cauliflower	Cabbage	Corn	Cucumbers
Celery	Cucumbers	Eggplant	Grapes
Citrus	Greens	Lima beans	Greens
Eggplant	Onions	Peaches	Pears
Mushrooms	Snap peas	Peas (Southern)	Squash (Summer)
Sweet potatoes	Strawberries	Watermelon	Tomatoes

Name   Date

Region 5

MS, MO, AR, LA, OK

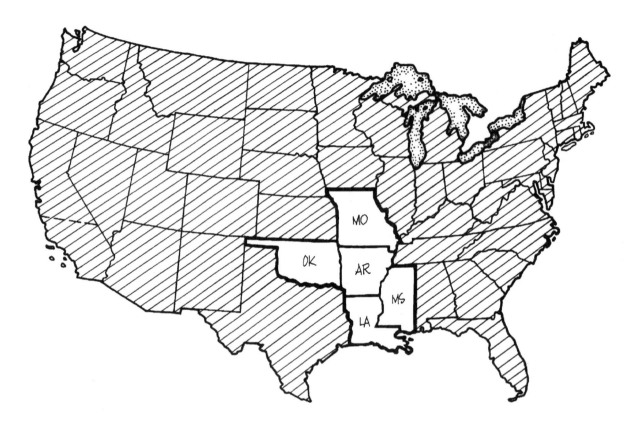

WINTER	SPRING	SUMMER	FALL
Apples	Asparagus	Blueberries	Cauliflower
Broccoli	Cauliflower	Corn	Eggplant
Cabbage	Corn	Lima beans	Grapes
Potatoes	Greens	Okra	Green beans
Spinach	Kale	Peppers (Hot,	Greens
Squash (Winter)	Kohlrabi	Sweet)	Pears
Sweet potatoes	Peas	Plums	Squash (Summer,
Turnips	Radishes	Tomatoes	Winter)
		Zucchini	Sweet potatoes

BECOMING FOOD SCIENTISTS : PLANTS : FOOD WEBS : AGRICULTURE : MAKING CHOICES

Name   Date

Region 6

TX, NM, AZ, CA (southern)

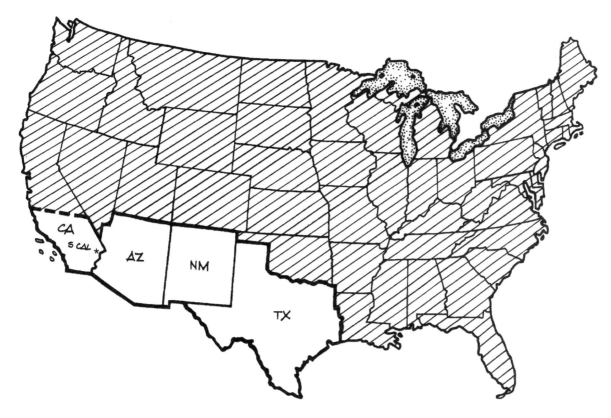

WINTER	SPRING	SUMMER	FALL
Beets	Broccoli	Asparagus	Artichokes
Carrots	Dates	Avocados	Greens
Cauliflower	Green beans	Cherries	Kiwis
Citrus	Greens	Corn	Peaches
Greens	Mushrooms	Cucumbers	Peppers (Hot,
Mushrooms	Oranges	Eggplant	Sweet)
Spinach	Raspberries	Figs	Persimmons
Squash (Winter)	Strawberries	Tomatoes	Squash (Summer,
			Winter)
			Sweet potatoes

*Changes in climate, even within regions, may result in changes in seasonal availability or harvest times of some foods.

Name	Date

Region 7

OH, IN, IL, IA, NE, KS

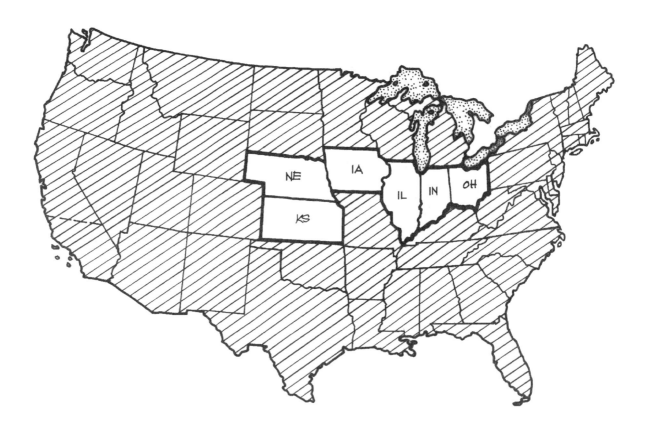

WINTER	SPRING	SUMMER	FALL
Apples CS	Asparagus	Beets	Apples
Cabbage CS	Greens	Cantaloupe	Broccoli
Garlic CS	Peas	Cauliflower	Carrots
Onions CS	Radishes	Corn	Greens
Potatoes CS	Rhubarb	Eggplant	Okra
Pumpkins CS	Spinach	Peppers (Hot,	Peas
Squash (Winter) CS	Sprouts	Sweet)	Raspberries (late)
Sweet potatoes CS	Strawberries	Tomatoes	Sweet potatoes
		Watermelon	

CS (cold storage): These are stored after harvest for use in multiple seasons.

LESSON 17: REGIONAL EATING

Name   Date

Region 8

CO, WY, UT, NV

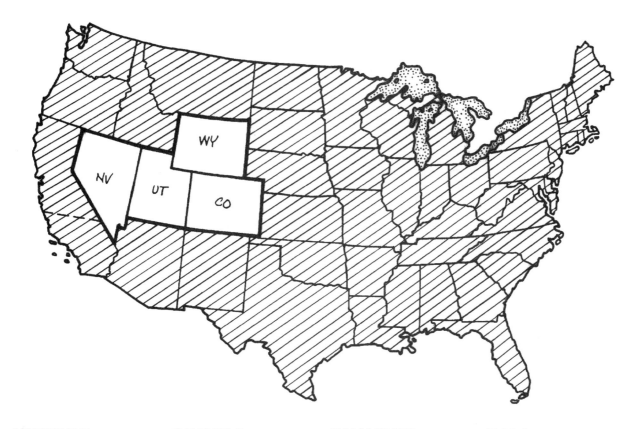

WINTER	SPRING	SUMMER	FALL
Apples CS	Arugula	Apricots	Broccoli
Beets CS	Asparagus	Beets	Cabbage
Cabbage CS	Carrots	Corn	Cauliflower
Carrots CS	Lettuce	Cucumbers	Eggplant
Onions CS	Onions	Peas	Peaches
Parsnips CS	Potatoes	Peppers (Hot, Sweet)	Pumpkin
Potatoes CS	Rhubarb	Raspberries	Spinach
Squash (Winter) CS	Spinach	Squash (Summer)	Tomatoes

CS (cold storage): These are stored after harvest for use in multiple seasons.

| Name | Date |

BECOMING FOOD SCIENTISTS : PLANTS : FOOD WEBS : AGRICULTURE : **MAKING CHOICES**

Bringing It Home

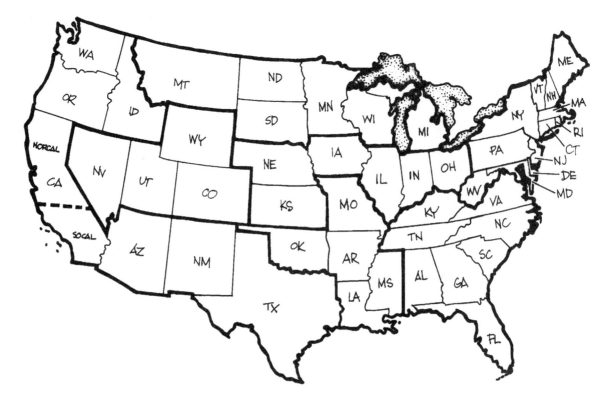

What Have You Learned?

Why is eating locally good for the environment and good for your health and the health of your community? Write a letter to a family member or friend who lives in another region telling them what's available in their region in different seasons. Explain the reasons for eating locally and seasonally and give them suggestions for how to get started.

Applying What You Learned

In class we talked about some of the ways you might take what you have learned about eating locally and make some changes in your life, your family's life, and your community that would help you move toward eating more locally grown food. Listed below are some of those actions. Your job is to pick two that you can do or start to do over the next few days. Of course you can do more if you want to! And if you have a suggestion that's not listed that you want to try, just let your teacher know.

• Choose a food from the seasonal list that you did not recognize and research what it is. Present your findings to the class. If the food is in season, bring it in for the class to observe or taste.

(continued on next page)

LESSON 17: REGIONAL EATING

Name	Date

Bringing It Home

- Challenge yourself and your family to spend $10 on locally grown food every week for a few months. Report on how hard or easy it is and why.

- Challenge yourself and your family to eat one meal a week that is made with all local ingredients. Report to the class how it goes.

- Challenge yourself and your family to eat a local fruit or vegetable every day for a month.

- Join your local Community Supported Agriculture program.

- Help your teacher organize a field trip to a local farm.

- Help your teacher organize a dinnertime "harvest party" and involve your families to teach them about local foods too.

- Create a cookbook made up of yummy recipes that use local, seasonal produce. You can do this by yourself or with the help of your friends and your teacher.

BECOMING FOOD SCIENTISTS : PLANTS : FOOD WEBS : AGRICULTURE : **MAKING CHOICES**

Comparing Farming Practices

AIM

To learn the advantages and disadvantages of different kinds of farming practices.

SCIENTIFIC PROCESSES

- **build theories, explain, contrast, debate**

OBJECTIVES:

Students will be able to:

- **identify issues related to farming;**

- **develop their own opinions concerning some issues related to farming practices;**

- **discuss and debate the advantages and disadvantages of different kinds of farming practices.**

OVERVIEW

In this lesson, students further their understanding of farming and farming methods. The student readings discuss industrial and sustainable farming practices. Drawing on what they have learned from the readings in this unit, students communicate what they have learned to a broader audience. In a teacher note, we offer some suggestions for projects your students might do to share this information. This activity offers students an opportunity to become reporters: to learn about a topic and report it to the public. Depending on the project format you and your class select, this lesson can be as simple or as complex as you choose to make it. The topic itself is complex, as it includes history, science, and technology. One goal of this lesson is to help students see how technology reflects and shapes the way humans have interacted with the environment over time. If students are struggling with some of the concepts presented in this module, you may wish to keep the project simple and focused on this unit's question.

MATERIALS

For the teacher:
- *Farm Web Sites* lesson resource
- *Agriculture and Ecosystems* teacher note
- *Farming Methods Project Tips* teacher note

For the class:
- (Optional) Sample newspapers, newsletters, or time lines for reference
- Chart paper
- Markers

For each student:
- (Optional) *Classroom Crops* student readings (pp. 161–184)
- (Optional) *Soil Particles* student reading (p. 198)
- (Optional) *Changing Weather Conditions* student reading (pp. 203–205)
- *Managing the Landscape* student reading
- *Farming Methods* student reading
- LiFE Log

PROCEDURE

Before You Begin:

- Review the *Agriculture and Ecosystems* and *Farming Methods Project Tips* teacher notes.

- Gather examples of different newspapers, newsletters, and time lines.

- (Optional) Remind students to bring in their student readings from Lessons 13, 15, and 16. These readings will provide more information for students to draw from as they develop their project.

- Make enough copies of the *Managing the Landscape* and *Farming Methods* student readings to distribute to each student.

- Make several copies of the *Farm Web Sites* lesson resources for students to use.

- If you have not already done so, post the Module Question and the Unit 5 Question at the front of the class.

MODULE QUESTION

How does nature provide us with food?

UNIT QUESTION

How can we use the science we've learned to make food and agriculture choices?

1. Review Module and Unit Questions

Review the Module and Unit questions with students. Explain that in this lesson they are going to learn about different kinds of farming practices. Using what they have learned in this unit, students will design a project, such as a newsletter, a bulletin-board display, or a debate, to share with other classes at school.

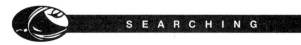

2. Discuss Theme of Project

The theme of this project is farming and farming practices: how we interact with nature to meet our needs. The audience for the project is the students' peers. This is an opportunity for your class to share what they have learned with others at your school.

Brainstorm with students a list of possible projects. Some possibilities include: a newsletter, an annotated time line, a bulletin-board display, a debate, a PowerPoint or other computer-generated presentation, or articles to submit to the school newspaper. Consider discussing this project with your students' language arts teacher. This may be a great opportunity to integrate science and language arts.

3. Research and Report

Distribute the student readings. After students have read through them, engage the class in a discussion about the project. Invite students to brainstorm ideas about what information they want to share. Accept all suggestions and record them on the chart paper. If you choose to make this a whole-class project, reach a consensus about the project content and approach. If you choose to have students work in small groups or pairs, make sure there are enough topics for everyone to participate.

Work with students to outline a project plan. Define specific tasks and assign them or ask for volunteers. If several students want to work on the same task, encourage them to work as a team. Help them assign responsibilities so all team members are active contributors. Consider establishing project benchmarks to track student progress.

4. Produce Project

Once all the student contributions are complete, assemble the projects and plan for how you will display or present the projects to the school community.

5. Summarize and Reflect

Discuss the project. Elicit from students what they have learned about industrial and sustainable farming. Have students respond to the following in their LiFE Logs: *What have you learned about farming? How do industrial farming practices differ from sustainable farming practices? Which type of farming practice is most like working with nature? What is your evidence?* If the students' project takes several days, have them make daily entries in their LiFE Logs documenting the development of the project and how they have synthesized what they have learned in the module each step of the way.

Farm Web Sites

Have students use these Web sites to help them with their project research.

- *www.agclassroom.org/gan/timeline/life_farm.htm*

  Ag in the Classroom's "A History of American Agriculture" offers two ways to search: by decade or by category, such as farm machinery and technology, life on a farm, or programs and policy.

- *www.historylink101.com/lessons/farm-city/story-of-farming.htm*

  Eric Rymer's world history Web site includes the history of farming. The site offers royalty-free photos of farms that students can use in their presentations.

- *www.connerprairie.org/historyonline/agimp.html*

  The Conner Prairie Living History Museum's site has photos and information about farm tools used in the 1800s.

- *www.ars.usda.gov/is/graphics/photos/*

  This USDA site is a source of high-quality digital images of fruit, vegetables, plants, crops, and much more.

- *www.wisconsinhistory.org*

  The Wisconsin Historical Society site includes a searchable database of historical pictures, including images of agricultural implements.

Agriculture and Ecosystems

Human society depends on agriculture. Since the origins of agriculture more than 10,000 years ago, human beings have become more and more dependent on a system in which a few people feed the rest of the population. This system helped support the development of a society in which people freed from raising food could do other tasks. Agriculture made it possible for people to settle down in groups that grew increasingly larger. Over thousands of years, new industries developed to meet society's needs. People looked for ways to help reduce labor needs and increase food production. New technologies were developed. Some technology made it possible to transport food over long distances without having it spoil. Some technology made it possible to convert dry, nonfertile land into productive agricultural fields. Some made it possible to eradicate pests and weeds quickly and efficiently. Until fairly recently, all of this progress seemed desirable.

As scientists have learned more about the way nature works, concerns have surfaced about the effects of agriculture. Think about a natural ecosystem and then compare it to agriculture, a manipulated ecosystem. Humans allow the species (crops) they favor to survive and do everything possible to remove the competition, such as pests and weeds. Yet by promoting monocropping, the growth of one crop in a concentrated area, farmers create a landscape where all the food resources the pests require are located in one spot and their populations can increase with very little effort.

To maximize crop production, fields are generally cleared as soon as the harvest is completed. In a natural ecosystem, plant material decays and the decomposition cycle eventually returns inorganic nutrients to the soil. Without decomposition, soils become depleted. To prevent this, synthetic fertilizers were developed, which required other resources. These chemicals can also run off fields and pollute water.

Concerns like these, as well as others, have made scientists and farmers look for ways to work with Nature rather than compete against her. It's a slow process. Now that we are aware of the effects of some of our interactions with nature, we need to consider the long-term impact of any proposed solution. What may appear beneficial today may have long-term negative effects that no one could even imagine. It's important to remember that many of the technologies we now view as detrimental to the environment were once seen as positive steps that were being taken to solve problems.

Farming Methods Project Tips

This lesson offers a great opportunity for students to demonstrate their understanding of how humans interact with nature to meet our food needs. Students can use readings from other lessons in this module as well as original research to prepare presentations that reflect their understanding of the topic. You may wish to discuss this project with your students' language arts and social studies teachers.

The project can take many forms. For example, it could combine visual material and text to create a time line of farming methods and technology. Creating a time line lets students bring together information from the extended history of agriculture. It is an excellent way to help students visualize the changes that have taken place in agriculture over time, and connect these changes to other significant social and cultural events. The lesson resource is a list of Web sites where students can research the history of agriculture and find royalty-free images.

Your students may enjoy creating a class newspaper and using this medium to share their knowledge. Consider having students use computer technology to create and produce a newsletter to distribute to the school community. Have students use the Internet to locate photographs and information to include in their newsletter. Some topics they might want to cover include reasons to eat locally, a feature story about sustainable agriculture, the top five reasons to support sustainable agriculture, or how technology affects the way we interact with nature.

Another project idea is to construct a chart that lists a specific technology, its designed purpose, and whether it reflects an industrial method or a more sustainable one. Charts can also be used to compare and contrast different farming methods, citing the advantages and disadvantages of each.

If your students have strong verbal skills, think about having them participate in a debate focusing on the positive and negative effects technological innovations have had on agriculture and the environment. Or they can write an organized, persuasive essay supporting a particular approach to farming.

Getting the Information

Collect information using different types of primary and secondary sources such as charts, newspapers, magazines, other media, museums, the Internet, and reference works.

Using the Information

Once students have the information, have them organize information from primary and secondary sources, identify the main ideas and supportive elements, evaluate information, differentiate fact from opinion, and identify differences and similarities in information.

Presenting the Information

If students are giving oral presentations, have them develop notes or memory aids, and remind groups to have everyone participate.

Name   Date

Managing the Landscape

How is a farm different from a natural ecosystem? Plants grow on a farm and plants grow in nature. Humans make the difference.

A farmer decides what plants to grow and controls the resources the plants get. Farmers also control some of the food-web interactions — from pest control to decomposition. Think about it. If pests attack a crop, farmers will use pest control. Once the crop is harvested, the fields are cleared of the dead plant material so a new crop can be planted. If the growing season is dry, farmers irrigate. If the soil is nutrient-poor, farmers add fertilizers.

Farmers decide what **technology** to use for their work. Technology, in this case, means more than computers. It includes any tool, machine, or technique that humans use to help them do work or complete a task.

Tools

This group includes shovels, hoes, watering cans, hoses, and any other kind of device that a person operates or uses. These simple tools are used in planting seeds and caring for plants. They are used most often when small amounts of food are being grown.

Machines

Animals, like horses or oxen, and engines supply the power for this type of technology. It includes tractors, **combines** (machines that help with harvesting), manure spreaders, and other machines that farmers drive through their fields. These machines help with many tasks, including preparing soil, planting seeds, spreading compost or fertilizer, and harvesting crops. Most of the time, the machines are powered by fossil fuels, such as gasoline or diesel fuel.

(continued on next page)

Name   Date

Managing the Landscape

Techniques

Sometimes farmers plant a crop that needs more nutrients than already exist in the soil. To change the soil, they add compost, manure, or commercially prepared synthetic fertilizer. Farmers also may need to control pests. The two basic kinds of pests are plant pests, or weeds, that compete with crops for nutrients and resources like water; and animal pests, like insects, rabbits, and deer, that eat the crops before they can be harvested. Farmers use fences to help protect crops from some pests. Some farmers use synthetic **insecticides** to control insect pests and synthetic **herbicides** to control weeds.

For more than 10,000 years, humans have used technology to help them plant seeds, care for their crops, and harvest them. Over time, the technology changed as people invented new ways to get work done faster and more easily. From digging sticks to animal-drawn plows to huge tractors pulling heavy equipment, as the technology developed, it changed the way people interacted with the natural world.

Name   Date

Farming Methods

Guiding Questions

- *What are some of the differences between industrial agriculture and sustainable agriculture?*

- *Why do some farmers prefer to use the industrial method?*

- *Why do some farmers prefer to use sustainable practices?*

- *What are three key features farmers use with industrial agriculture?*

- *What are three key features farmers use with sustainable agriculture?*

In this lesson, you will learn about two different kinds of farming systems in the United States. Some farmers practice a method known as **industrial agriculture.** These are large farms that specialize in **monocropping,** or growing one crop. This type of farming concentrates on maximizing production to make the most profit. This approach sees nature as a competitor and tries to control it. The other, very different farming method is **sustainable agriculture.** This is often practiced on smaller farms that grow different kinds of crops that can be sold throughout the year. Sustainable farming practices are an attempt to try to work with nature. In this reading, you will learn about these two very different kinds of farming and some of the advantages and disadvantages of each method.

(continued on next page)

Name	Date

Farming Methods

Industrial Farming

This drawing shows an example of industrial farming. Sometimes this approach is called **agribusiness.** Sometimes the people who own the farm do not live there and do not work on the farm. Often the owners consider this a business, and the product they make is food. This approach to farming uses all available technology in order to maximize harvests and minimize the costs of human labor. Three key features of industrial farming are the use of large farm machines, the use of synthetic fertilizers, and the use of synthetic pesticides.

People who use this approach to farming think of themselves as competing against nature. They use methods that help them control nature. Notice that the farm worker is using a large irrigation system to water a field that is planted with only one type of crop. The irrigation system is set up to work automatically, on a schedule. By automating some of the tasks, the owner can reduce the number of people who work on the field, which will increase his profits. Another farm worker is using a large tractor to work the field.

This method of farming is physically easier, since heavy machinery does much of the work. Farm workers don't have to use their own energy to prepare fields for planting, sowing seeds, watering crops, or harvesting them. One person can farm a larger area

(continued on next page)

Name   Date

Farming Methods

and produce more food for less money, which will increase his profits when he takes the food to market. Using synthetic fertilizers, the farm workers can make sure that plants are getting exactly the nutrients they want to give them, in exactly the amount the plant needs. Using synthetic pesticides means that the farm workers can reduce the crop damage due to pests, which will increase the farm owner's profits.

Food grown this way is often less expensive than food grown using sustainable practices. Industrial farming requires less farm labor, which reduces the cost of producing the food.

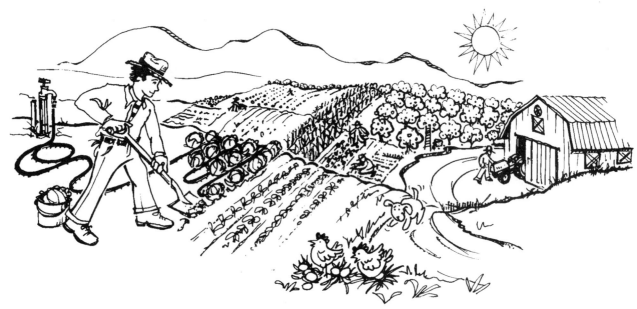

Sustainable Agriculture

This drawing shows an example of sustainable farming practices. This type of farming uses more human labor to produce food than industrial farming does. The farmers are growing crops in a way that helps support a healthy soil ecosystem and works with nature. The key features of this approach to farming are the use of small machines or people to do the work, the use of compost and manure as fertilizer, and the use of natural methods for pest control.

Notice that the farm family in the drawing is growing different kinds of crops, including a fruit orchard. This is called **diversified farming.** The reason for growing different crops is to support the farm family with a variety of crops so that it doesn't depend on

(continued on next page)

238

Name   Date

Farming Methods

just one. This practice of growing more than one crop protects farmers if they have bad weather. For example, there may be too much rain or there may be not enough rain for a crop to produce a good harvest. Farmers can rely on other crops grown at other times to get them through the year. Planting different kinds of crops also mimics the diversity in nature's ecosystems and makes it easier to use natural methods as a way to control pests and fertilize crops.

Sustainable agriculture also uses crop rotation. This means that different crops are planted on the same land in different years. For example, if a farmer plants tomato plants on a field one year, the next year he will plant a different kind of crop on that same field. This practice helps maintain good soil conditions and helps with pest control.

To support healthy soil, sustainable farming uses composting as an alternative to inorganic, synthetic fertilizers. Farmers also use **green manures,** which are crops that are grown with the specific purpose of turning them into the soil. Green manure adds nutrients and organic matter to keep the soil ecosystem healthy.

Sustainability means thinking about our children's children. It means meeting our needs today without compromising the ability of future generations to meet their needs. These practices try to preserve the environment. Farmers still make a profit, but not at the expense of the land.

Farmer Frieda's Design Project

AIM

To use what we have learned about agriculture to design a farm.

SCIENTIFIC PROCESSES

• **question, search, apply**

OBJECTIVES

Students will be able to:

• **appreciate how much work it takes to be a farmer and how farms work;**

• **understand what happens on a diversified farm during the growing season;**

• **apply what they have learned to design an imaginary farm.**

OVERVIEW

Thus far, students have been exploring the Unit 5 Question, *How can we use the science we learned to make food and agriculture choices?* In this unit, students are studying the world of agriculture and the role humans play in producing the foods we eat. This lesson provides students with an opportunity to pull together their understanding of what happens on a working farm. In this lesson, students design an imaginary farm for Farmer Frieda. Students read about what Frieda wants to grow on her diversified pizza and salad farm, including salad greens, tomatoes, onions, and herbs. As homework, students write descriptions in their LiFE Logs of their ideal pizza farm by choosing which ingredients to grow on their farms and describing what their lives would be like if they were pizza farmers.

MATERIALS

For the class:
• (Optional) Magazines with photographs of farms or large vegetable gardens

For each team:
• A collection of all the student readings for this module
• Several sheets of chart paper
• Markers and pencils

For each student:
• *Design-a-Farm Project* activity sheet
• LiFE Log

PROCEDURE

Before You Begin:

- Make enough copies of the *Design-a-Farm Project* activity sheet to distribute to each student.

- Gather together a collection of all the student readings for this module for each design team. You may prefer to have students bring in their own copies of the readings.

- Gather images of farms or large vegetable gardens for students to use as reference for their design project.

- If you have not already done so, post the Module Question and the Unit 5 Question at the front of the class.

MODULE QUESTION

How does nature provide us with food?

UNIT QUESTION

How can we use the science we've learned to make food and agriculture choices?

1. Review Module and Unit Questions

Review the Module and Unit questions with students. Explain that in this lesson they are going to design a farm. To do this, they will need to pull together all the information they have learned about how nature provides us with food.

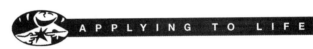
SEARCHING

2. Discuss Design Project

Distribute the student reading to each student. Review the information on the sheet. Remind students that Farmer Frieda is the client for this project and they need to remember what her needs are. Elicit from students what the design requirements are for Frieda's farm. *What does Frieda want you to do? Does it matter to Frieda what kind of farm you design? What crops does Frieda want to grow? Does she need to make money? How much land does she have? What else does Frieda want? How much time is there before next year's festival?*

APPLYING TO LIFE

3. Create Design Teams

Divide the class into small groups. Have each team elect a team leader to guide the project and keep track of the details and deadlines. Help teams identify tasks and make assignments. Have team leaders record this information on a chart. Some students may want to work on the marketing while others work on the farm design. Encourage and support collaborative work.

4. Organize Project Work

Meet with team leaders to discuss project deadlines and to schedule presentations for the end of each stage of the design. Check each team's progress. If necessary, adjust deadlines.

5. Present and Critique Projects

Invite each design team to display its project. Ask each team leader to discuss the team's project design, why the team chose this particular design solution to Frieda's "problem," and why the team thinks Frieda should choose its design. Invite the team's marketing person or group to present its strategy.

Ask the design teams to critique each other's projects. They should explain what they like about the project's approach and what they think doesn't work, and why. Remind students that any criticism should be offered as constructive criticism.

After all the teams have presented their designs, congratulate them on their fine solutions. Consider keeping the designs on display and inviting other classes to view the work.

6. Homework

As homework, ask students to write descriptions in their LiFE Logs of their ideal pizza farm. This time they are the farmers and they can choose which ingredients to grow on their farms. Ask students to write several paragraphs describing what their lives would be like if they were pizza farmers.

Name   Date

Design-a-Farm Project

You have just won a chance to design a farm for Farmer Frieda. Frieda decided she wanted to grow the crops to make a pizza because she loves pizza. Plus, she lives near Pizzatown, and each fall, the town holds a huge pizza and salad festival. It's a great chance for Frieda to show everyone how wonderful and tasty the food is that she grows. This is a great opportunity for you to think about all that you have learned about food, farming technology, and the environment. You also get to make a pitch for supporting local farmers. It's very exciting and you're ready to drop everything and start plowing the fields and planting the crops. But wait, there are a couple of things you need to think about:

1. Everyone in Pizzatown is counting on local farmers to provide all the tomatoes, herbs, and salad greens for their pizza and salad festival at the end of the summer. Frieda needs to provide enough tomatoes and salad ingredients to feed 25 people. The festival estimates that they will need one pizza for every two people. Frieda's recipe for fresh-tomato-and-herbs pizza topping calls for three ripe tomatoes and one-half cup fresh, chopped herbs, like parsley, chives, or basil, for each pizza.

2. Frieda's not sure which kind of farm she wants. She's counting on you to come up with a good design. Should it be a diversified farm or an industrial model? For Frieda, farming is her way to support herself and her family, so she needs to make money. But she also cares about the environment. She's not sure what to do and wants you to use your expertise to advise her.

   There are so many details to think about, and right now all Frieda can focus on is the festival and the deadline. She needs to have great produce for the festival and it's only 11 months away! She wants lots of great-tasting tomatoes and onions and huge baskets full of herbs like basil and oregano. Plus, she wants salad greens, cucumbers, chives, radishes, parsley, cilantro, peppers, borage, and dill for the salad and salad dressing.

3. Pizzatown is leasing Frieda a three-acre lot at the edge of town. There's a barn there where Frieda can store her equipment. There's even a place for a small tractor. A stream runs near the property. Plus, there is lots of sun and very little shade.

4. One of the citizens of Pizzatown knew there was going to be a contest and decided to help out. She and her family started hundreds of seedlings in her greenhouse. She has said Frieda can have as many seedlings as she has room for. This is very good news.

(continued on next page)

Name	Date

Design-a-Farm Project

Here are some tips to help guide your work. This is a big project, so think about dividing the work into four separate stages.

Stage One: Type of Farm

• What type of farm will you design? What farming practices will you recommend?

• What technology will Frieda need?

• Where can you find the information you need to plan the farm? *Hint:* Look back at the student readings in this module.

• What kinds of jobs are involved in growing plants?

• What happens on a farm through the different seasons of the year?

Stage Two: Planting Analysis

• What kind of plants will Frieda grow? Think about the ingredients you need for a salad. What about the pizza? You know you want tomatoes, but what else do you want? Basil, onions, garlic, oregano, parsley? Anything else? Make a list of all the plants Frieda will grow for the salad and all the plants she will grow for the pizza.

• How many of each plant will she need to grow? How much room will you need to plan for each crop? Remember, Frieda needs to grow enough salad ingredients to feed 25 people and enough tomatoes, onions, and basil to make pizza topping for 13 pizzas. To make sure she has enough to make the pizza, Frieda wants to plant 50 tomato plants, 30 basil plants, 40 onions, 10 oregano plants, 10 parsley plants, and some garlic, if there is room. She said you can include other plants for the pizza, too. It's up to you. It is also up to you to decide how many of each type of plant you are using in the salad you want to grow. Make a list of plants and the number of each you need to grow.

• For each plant, make a list of what that plant needs to grow and survive. Remember to include nonliving things.

(continued on next page)

Name	Date

Design-a-Farm Project

- Are there pests that might destroy your crops? What can you do to prevent this?

- What else do you need to consider for your plants?

Stage Three: Drawing

You will probably need to do a few rough drafts before you start on your final draft. Consult with fellow designers. Your final draft should have dimensions of the fields, interior and exterior views of the barn, and labels for each part of the farm.

Stage Four: Marketing

Frieda heard that some of your design-team members once worked in advertising. She wants you to help her design some marketing tools to help her convince others about the importance of eating locally grown food and supporting local farmers, especially Frieda! First of all, she needs a name for her farm. Once she has a name, she'd like to put it on a poster or a banner for her farm stand or to display at the festival. She also thought about designing a T-shirt to advertise her products.

- What kind of name do you think Frieda should use for her farm? She wants it to be easy to remember. She's not sure if it should be funny, cute, or serious. She thought about "Pizzatown Produce," or "Herbs, Etcetera," or even "Frieda's Pizza Farm." She hopes you have some ideas.

- What kind of advertising catches your eye? Remember, the products you are promoting are food and local farmers.

- What makes you want to buy one kind of food rather than another? Consider interviewing some adults to hear what they have to say.

- Think about the different ways that advertisers get their messages to you. Is music important? How about color? Do words rhyme?

Be sure to keep notes on all the references you used. Frieda wants to know where you got all of your information.

Bringing It All Together

AIM

To reflect on and synthesize what we have learned in this module about growing food.

SCIENTIFIC PROCESSES

- **construct knowledge, put into action**

OBJECTIVES

Students will be able to:

- **express in writing and drawing an answer to the Module Question, *How does nature provide us with food?*;**

- **evaluate changes in their understanding of how nature provides us with food;**

- **create a list of food-choice guidelines based on what they have learned;**

- **describe why each of their guidelines is important.**

OVERVIEW

This final lesson in the module is an opportunity for you and your students to contemplate, synthesize, and establish how students' answers to the Module Question, *How does nature provide us with food?* have changed. To do this, the students repeat some of what they did in Lesson 4. Students add to or redraw their visual representation of how nature provides us with food. Next, they discuss the ways in which what they learned in this module has influenced their food choices. From this they develop a list of food-choice guidelines — rules or concepts — that they would like to follow now and in the future. The module ends with students answering the Module Question in their LiFE Logs. After students answer the question, they compare what they wrote today with what they wrote when they answered the Module Question in Lesson 4. As a class, they discuss how their answers changed and they write a paragraph that describes their individual changes.

MATERIALS

For the teacher:
- *Food-Choice Guidelines* lesson resource

For the class:
- Chart paper
- Markers

For each student:
- Large index cards
- Markers or crayons
- Food-production picture drawn in Lesson 4
- LiFE Log

PROCEDURE

Before You Begin:

- Ask students to review the pictures they drew in Lesson 4 that reflected their understanding of how nature provides us with food.

- Review the *Food-Choice Guidelines* lesson resource.

- Be sure you have the Module Question and all five Unit questions posted at the front of the classroom.

MODULE QUESTION

How does nature provide us with food?

UNIT QUESTION

How can we use the science we've learned to make food and agriculture choices?

 THEORIZING

1. Review the Module Question and All Unit Questions

If you have not already done so, post the Module Question and the questions from Units 1–5 in front of the classroom. Explain to students that this is the final lesson in the module, and it is an opportunity to reflect and synthesize what they have learned. They will think about the answer to the Module Question and how studying the Unit questions helped them expand their answer to the Module Question.

2. Create a Picture

Ask students to draw a picture on an index card that represents how nature provides us with food. Remind students that they did this same activity in Lesson 4. Encourage students to include new things that they have learned in this module in their pictures. Remind students to use diagrams, words, and arrows in their representation of how nature provides us with food.

3. Share Pictures

After students have finished drawing, invite them to share their work with the class. Encourage students to be supportive of each other throughout the questioning and discussion of what was learned. You may want to use these pictures to replace the pictures students drew in Lesson 4 and keep them posted in the classroom.

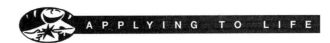 **APPLYING TO LIFE**

4. Develop Food-Choice Guidelines

Explain that now students are going to think about guidelines they can use when they choose what food to eat based on what they have learned in the module. First, ask them to share any ways this module has changed what they eat. *Does anyone shop at farmers' markets now? Does anyone try to eat foods just as they came from the farm? Does anyone try to choose foods grown organically? Anything else you do differently?*

Define food-choice guidelines as rules or concepts one would use when trying to decide what to eat. Ask students to share guidelines they might now try to use when making food choices based on what they have learned in this module. Create a list of their guidelines on chart paper. For each guideline, have the class develop a reason for the guideline, under the heading "why this guideline is important." See the lesson resource for a sample list of guidelines. Conclude this discussion with concrete references to how these guidelines can be followed, such as reviewing locations of farmers' markets and community gardens.

5. LiFE Logs

Have students write an answer to the Module Question, *How does nature provide us with food?* They can use their picture as a guide. Encourage students to write as complete an answer to the Module Question as they can. Remind them to look at and think about the Unit questions and to incorporate what they learned in each unit, especially Units 2–5, into their answer to the Module Question. Refer to the **Assessment** section of the introduction for more information on assessing your students' learning.

6. Reflect on What They Learned

After students complete their answer to the Module Question, have them compare what they wrote now to what they wrote during Lesson 4. Ask students to write a short paragraph that describes how their answer has changed. Have some students read their current answers to the Module Question. Ask students to share what they have learned. Encourage students to continue to think about and apply what they have learned by following the food-choice guidelines just developed and talking about food-production issues with family and friends.

Food-Choice Guidelines

This is a sample of the types of food-choice guidelines that students may develop. They may have other ideas not represented here. This is fine. If students don't think of some of the ideas in these sample guidelines, present these ideas and ask students if they want to add them to their list.

GUIDELINE	WHY IT IS IMPORTANT
Eat more food from plants, and less food from animals.	When we eat plants (producers) we are getting the sun's energy more directly, so less energy is "lost" than when we eat animals (consumers) that eat plants.
Buy food from local farmers whenever possible.	This helps keep local farms in business and less energy is used to transport food. The food is also fresher and may be more nutritious.
Shop at farmers' markets and/or join a Community Supported Agriculture program (CSA).	This is a great way to directly support local farmers.
Eat food from all different parts of the plant.	This will help us get the nutrients we need, and it can make eating more fun and interesting.
Eat more foods that come directly from plants or animals and less food that has been changed or processed.	This gives us the nutrients we need, helps farmers, and less energy is used to process food.
Compost food scraps whenever possible.	This helps return nutrients to the soil and decreases waste.
Grow some of your own food.	This will help increase appreciation of farmers, is lots of fun, and is a wonderful way to get excited about trying new foods — plus the food tastes great.
Join a community garden or grow herbs in your home.	These are some easy ways to grow some of our own food.
Don't waste food.	Farmers grow all the food we eat. Even processed, packaged foods are made from ingredients grown by farmers. Natural resources and farmers' time and effort are used to grow our food.

Bibliography

American Association for the Advancement of Science. 1993. *Benchmarks for scientific literacy.* New York: Oxford University Press.

Anderson, C., Sheldon, W., & DuBay, E. 1990. The effects of instruction on college nonmajors' conceptions of respiration and photosynthesis. *Journal of Research in Science Teaching, 27 (8),* 761–76.

Ausubel, D. 1968. *Educational psychology: A cognitive view,* New York: Holt, Rinehart, & Winston.

Corn Refiners Association. 2005. Retrieved January 5, 2005, from *www.corn.org.*

Driver, R., Squires, A., Rushworth, P., & Wood-Robinson, V. 1994. *Making sense of secondary science: Research into children's ideas.* London/New York: Routledge.

Goh, N., Yoke-Kum, W., & Lian-Sai, C. 1993. Simply photosynthesis. *Science and Children, 31 (1),* 32–34.

Hershey, D. 2004. *Avoid misconceptions when teaching about plants.* Retrieved September 21, 2005, from *www.actionbioscience.org.*

Kyle, W.C., & Shymansky, J.A. 1989. Enhancing learning through conceptual change teaching. *Research Matters — to the Science Teacher, 2.* Retrieved October 25, 2005, from *www.educ.sfu.ca/narstsite/publications/research/concept.htm.*

National Agricultural Statistics Service, USDA. 1997. Noncitrus Fruits and Nuts Preliminary Summary. Economic Research Service, USDA. Retrieved October 25, 2005, from *http://usda.mannlib.cornell.edu/reports/nassr/fruit/pnf-bb/ncit0198.txt.*

National Research Council (NRC). 1996. *National science education standards.* Washington, DC: National Academy Press.

Renner, J.W., Abraham, M.R., Grzybowski, E.B., & Marek, E.A. 1990. Understandings and misunderstandings of eighth graders of four physics concepts found in textbooks. *Journal of Research in Science Teaching, 27,* 35–54.

Roth, K.J. 2001. *Student-focused curriculum materials development: The "food for plants" story.* American Association for the Advancement of Science Conference on Developing Textbooks That Promote Science Literacy, February 27–March 2, 2001. Retrieved October 13, 2005, from *www.project2061.org/meetings/textbook/literacy/roth.htm.*

Schraer, W.D. & Stoltze, H.J. 1999. *Biology: The study of life, seventh edition.* Upper Saddle River, NJ: Prentice Hall Simon & Schuster Education Group.

Simply Recipe. 2005. [Grape-juice recipe.] Retrieved January 31, 2005, from *www.elise.com/recipes/archives/000107making_grape_juice.php.*

Stern, L. & Roseman, J. 2004. Can middle-school science textbooks help students learn important ideas? Findings from Project 2061's curriculum evaluation study: Life Science. *Journal of Research in Science Teaching, 41 (6),* 538–68.

Wilkins, J.L., Bowdish, E., & Sobal, J. 2002. Consumer perceptions of seasonal and local foods: A study in a US community. *Ecology of Food and Nutrition, 41 (5),* 415–39.

Web-Based Resources

Center for Ecoliteracy

www.ecoliteracy.org

This Web site offers extensive information about the Center's Rethinking School Lunch (RSL) program, including a downloadable guide that contains tools and creative solutions to the challenges of improving school lunch programs, academic performance, ecological knowledge, and the well-being of children.

Center for Science in the Public Interest (CSPI)

www.cspinet.org

Since 1971 CSPI has been a strong advocate for nutrition and health, food safety, alcohol policy, and sound science. Its award-winning newsletter, *Nutrition Action Healthletter*, is the largest-circulation health newsletter in North America, providing reliable information on nutrition and health.

Chefs Collaborative

www.chefscollaborative.org

This national network of more than 1,000 members of the food community promotes sustainable cuisine by celebrating the joys of local, seasonal, and artisanal cooking.

Community Food Security Coalition (CFSC)

www.foodsecurity.org

CFSC is a nonprofit North American organization dedicated to supporting sustainable, local, and regional food systems through education, advocacy, and networking. It helps communities create systems of growing, manufacturing, processing, making available, and selling regional, sustainable foods. CFSC has more than 325 member organizations.

Equal Exhange

www.equalexchange.com

This retail Web site offers a wide range of fair trade, gourmet products including coffee, tea, sugar, chocolate bars, and cocoa.

Fair Trade Certified

www.transfairusa.org/content/support/

Use this Web site to get involved and support fair trade goods. Spread the word to your friends, family, and co-workers. Learn how to change the world, starting with one cup of coffee.

Food Research Action Center (FRAC)

www.frac.org

This nonprofit organization works with public policy to end hunger and malnutrition in the United States. FRAC's Web site offers information about legislation, policy, news, and lobbying.

Food Routes Network (FRN)

www.foodroutes.org

FRN is a national nonprofit organization that provides communications tools, technical support, networking, and information resources to organizations nationwide that are working to rebuild local, community-based food systems. Its Web site includes resources for supporting local food and farmers.

Local Foods in the United Kingdom

www.localfoodworks.org

The local food team of the UK's Soil Association works to support local food and farmers in the UK. Its Web site offers news, information, networking, and CSA information.

Local Harvest

www.localharvest.org

Nothing tastes better than a tomato just picked from the garden. The freshest, healthiest, most flavorful organic food is what's grown closest to your home. Use the Local Harvest map to find all the farmers' markets, family farms, locally grown produce, grass-fed meats, and other sources of sustainably grown food in your area.

National Campaign for Sustainable Agriculture (NSCA)

www.sustainableagriculture.net

NCSA is dedicated to educating the public on the importance of a sustainable food and agriculture system that is economically viable, environmentally sound, socially just, and humane. Sign up for its action alert list to get involved in promoting a more sustainable food system.

National Gardening Association (NGA)

www.garden.org, www.kidsgardening.org

NGA's Web sites offer extensive horticultural information, how-to planting guides, networking opportunities for educators, grants and awards, the Adopt a School Garden™ program, and plant-based educational resources, curricula, and products.

Northeast Regional Food Guide

www.nutrition.cornell.edu/foodguide/archive/index.html

The Guide is a new nutrition education tool to help consumers in the Northeastern United States choose a nutritious diet that promotes health and supports an active life. In addition to these nutrition and health goals, the Guide encourages Northeasterners to eat foods grown in their region. It is available through the Cornell University Cooperative Extension.

Robin Van En Center for CSA Resources

www.csacenter.org

The Robyn Van En Center offers a variety of services to existing and new CSA farmers and shareholders nationally. It provides outreach and works to gain publicity for CSA farms in order to benefit community farmers and consumers. Use its Web site to locate a CSA or learn about other initiatives.

Slow Food

www.slowfood.com

This international association promotes food and wine culture, as well as agricultural biodiversity. Use its Web site to learn about events, publications, and to see how the rest of the world honors slow food.

Stone Barns Center for Food and Agriculture

www.stonebarnscenter.org

The Stone Barns Center is a nonprofit farm, educational center, and restaurant in Westchester County, New York. Visit this site to find out about the Center's student programs, teacher programs, farm camp, and learning resources, or to schedule a free visit to the farm.

The Food Project

www.thefoodproject.org

The Food Project works with youth and volunteers to grow food. It donates half the food to homeless shelters and sells the other half as a part of a CSA. In addition, it is a resource for farmers, organizations, and individuals.

The True Food Network

www.truefoodnow.org

This site provides information on genetically engineered foods. Click on the "shopper's guide" for a listing of products, including those that contain genetically engineered ingredients.

Vegetable Program U Mass Amherst

www.umassvegetable.org

Lots of information about farming in the Northeast and more information on CSAs.

Glossary

Abiotic — The nonliving elements found in an ecosystem, including air, rocks, sunshine, and water.

Agribusiness — Agriculture designed to generate profits and growth for corporate investors. Agribusiness decisions are made to maximize short-run profits and growth. Decisions are not made with a primary focus of meeting the long-term needs of society. (Contrast with **sustainable agriculture.**)

Air cavity — In a **seed**, the space between the **seed coat** and the **endosperm.**

Anther — In a flower, the top part of the male reproductive organs. It produces the pollen.

Biotic — The living elements found in an ecosystem, including plants, animals, and microbes.

Carnivore — An animal that eats only other animals.

Castings — The undigested food that a worm excretes as waste. The compost in worm bins is made up of worm castings.

Chemical energy — Energy that is contained within chemical bonds. The energy in a peanut is contained in the chemical bonds within the peanut.

Chlorophyll — The green pigment that gives plants their green color. Plants that are colors other than green also have chlorophyll, but they have other pigments that dominate the chlorophyll.

Chloroplast — The part of a plant cell that contains the green pigment **chlorophyll. Photosynthesis** takes place in the chloroplasts.

Clitellum — The reproductive structure in a worm. The clitellum is a band that forms in the middle of the worm's body. After the clitellum hardens it becomes a cocoon that the worm slides off its body. Each cocoon can hold up to 20 fertilized eggs. After about 3 weeks, the eggs hatch.

Combine — A machine for harvesting grains. In one operation it combines cutting, threshing, separation, and cleaning of grain, as well as dispersing the stems, stalks, or other crop residue.

Control group — In an experiment, the group that has the usual or normal conditions to compare to the **experimental group.** For example, in an experiment to determine what would happen to a plant that does not get sunlight, the control group would be plants that are exposed to sunlight. The experimental group would be plants that are not exposed to sunlight.

Crop — In a worm, the place where food is broken down into smaller pieces. Food can also be stored in the crop.

CSA (community supported agriculture) — In basic terms, a CSA consists of a community of individuals who pledge support to a farm operation so that the farmland becomes, either legally or spiritually, the community's farm, with the growers and consumers providing mutual support and sharing the risks and benefits of food production. Members or shareholders of the farm or garden pledge in advance to cover the anticipated costs of the farm operation and the farmer's salary. In return, they receive shares in the farm's bounty throughout the growing season, as well as satisfaction gained from reconnecting to the land. Members also share in risks, including poor harvests due to unfavorable weather or pests. (USDA definition)

Cuticle — In a **leaf,** a waxy, transparent layer that acts as a waterproof cover for the **epidermis.**

Decomposer — An organism that breaks down the remains of dead plants and animals. This process releases substances that can be reused by new plants.

Decomposition — The process of breaking down organic material, causing it to decay.

Detritivore — A multicellular organism, like a worm, insect, or nematode, that primarily eats decomposed plants or animals.

Detritus — The remains of a plant or animal that have been broken down or decomposed. Detritus is an important source of nutrients for plants and other living things.

Diversified farming — A method in which a farm grows a wide variety of crops and uses crop rotation. These farming techniques can make a farm more resilient to severe weather conditions or crop disease. On a diversified farm, farmers also tend to use more ecologically friendly methods to fertilize crops and control pests.

Embryo — The earliest stage of development of an animal or a plant.

Endosperm — A tissue found in the **seed** of flowering plants. Endosperm provides nutrition to the developing **embryo.** It is mostly composed of starch, though it can also contain oils and protein.

Energy — The ability to do **work.** The amount of energy a thing has predicts how much work it can do, or how much heat it can exchange.

Epidermis — In a **leaf,** the outer layer of protective cells.

Experimental design — The steps to conduct an experiment. These steps are also called the methods for the experiment. In an experiment, the **experimental group** is compared to the **control group.**

Experimental group — In an experiment, the group that is exposed to a condition that is being tested in order to determine the effects of the condition. For example, in an experiment to determine what would happen to a plant that does not get sunlight, the plants in the experimental group would be deprived of sunlight in order to determine the effects of this condition.

Flower — The reproductive organ in a plant. Its function is to produce **seeds.** After fertilization, a flower can develop into a **fruit** containing the seeds.

Food system — The process by which food is produced and made available to consumers. The steps in the food system include growing, harvesting, **preserving, processing, transporting, packaging,** storing, purchasing, consuming, and discarding waste.

Fruit — The ripened **ovary** of the plant. It contains the **seeds** of a flowering plant.

Germ — The part of a **seed** that will become the new plant when the seed is planted. The germ has a high oil content.

Gizzard — In a worm, the organ to which food travels after going through the **crop.** The gizzard has strong muscles that act like teeth to help break down the food. Sand in the gizzard helps chop up the food into even smaller pieces.

Global food system — A **food system** that is very complex and extends all over the world. Most American consumers purchase their food far away from where the food production and **processing** occurred. Consumers want the best quality at the lowest price, which results in moving food production to places where land and labor costs are low. Food is an international trade item. Recently there has been an increased interest in purchasing food from local farmers and reestablishing connections between consumers and farmers. (See **CSA.**)

Green manures — Crops that are grown with the specific intent of being plowed under, where they add nutrients and organic matter to the soil.

Guard cells — In a leaf, the cells that border the **stomata** and allow it to open and close, depending on conditions such as temperature or amount of carbon dioxide.

Healthy soil — Soil that contains organic matter. Soil is made mostly of inorganic matter—sand, silt, and clay. Although organic matter is just one component of soil, it is vital to making the soil healthy.

Heart — In a worm, five pairs of blood vessels that bring oxygen to all parts of the worm.

Herbicide — A chemical substance or living organism used to kill or control unwanted vegetation such as brush, weeds, and certain trees.

Herbivore — An animal that eats only plants.

Humus — A vital building block of soil that helps it retain water and nutrients. Humus is made up of naturally decomposed plant or animal remains. The term is often used synonymously with soil organic matter.

Hypothesis — An informed or educated prediction, or a guess, about the results of an experiment.

Industrial agriculture — Another term for **agribusiness.** (Contrast with **sustainable agriculture.**)

Insecticide — A synthetic or organic chemical used to kill or repel insects.

Intestine — In a worm, the organ where food travels after leaving the **gizzard.** Digestion is completed in the intestines.

Leaf — In a plant, a specialized organ for conducting **photosynthesis,** the process of converting light energy, water, and carbon dioxide into food energy.

Legumes — Edible **seeds** inside a pod. Well-known plants that bear legumes include alfalfa, clover, peas, beans, and peanuts.

Monocropping — Growing only one crop on the land. This method can lead to intensified pest pressure, which can result in increased pesticide use.

Mouth — In a worm, the opening through which food enters. The food travels from the mouth to the crop.

Omnivore — An animal that eats both plants and animals.

Ovary — In a **flower,** the bottom part of the female reproductive organs. It contains the **ovules,** or new **seeds.**

Ovule — In a **flower,** the **embryo** sac that develops into a **seed** after fertilization.

Packaging — Anything that keeps food contained. Usually made of cardboard, plastic, or glass, packaging protects our food, prevents contamination, and helps keep food fresh.

Palisade layer — Cells just below the top surface of a **leaf.** Most of the **chloroplasts** are in the palisade layer.

Peg — A **stem** that is formed from the **ovary** of a peanut plant. The peanut **embryo** is in the tip of the peg that grows downward, into the soil.

Petals — In a **flower,** the flat structures that are often brightly colored, showy, and fragrant. The petals surround and protect the reproductive organs.

Petiole — The **stalk** by which a **leaf** is attached to a **stem.** The part of the celery we eat is the petiole. It attaches the short, wide stem on the bottom of the celery stalk to the leaves that are on the top.

Phloem — A tissue in vascular plants, used to transport nutrients from the **leaves** to other parts of the plant.

Photo — A prefix for many words. It means "light."

Photosynthesis — The process by which plants absorb sunlight to make food. The plant uses the light energy, carbon dioxide from the air, and water from the soil to make sugars that are the plant's food.

Pistil — In a **flower,** the female reproductive organ. It is usually found in the center of the flower. It has three parts: the **stigma,** the **style,** and the **ovary.**

Pollinators — The agents that move pollen from the male **anthers** to the female **stigma** in order to fertilize the **ovule.** Bees are a widely recognized pollinator, but other insects, bats, and birds are also pollinators.

Preserving — Preparing food or any perishable substance so as to avoid **decomposition** or fermentation. Canned tomatoes are a preserved form of fresh tomatoes.

Processing — Preparing or putting food, or some material, through a prescribed procedure in manufacturing. For example, wheat berries are processed to make flour by grinding them; the flour and other ingredients are processed to make bread.

Producers — An organism that makes its own food from inorganic substances. Producers use light energy, water, and carbon dioxide to make sugars, which are their food. Plants are producers.

QuESTA Learning Cycle — A tool to frame the learning process for inquiry-based science. Includes five phases: Questioning, Experimenting, Searching, Theorizing, and Applying to Life.

Root — The part of a plant that takes in water and minerals from the soil and helps anchor the plant in the ground.

Scavenger — An animal that eats dead plants or animals. Scavengers help break down dead organic materials into smaller pieces. Examples are crows, vultures, cockroaches, and bald eagles.

Science inquiry — A method through which students think like scientists to: ask a testable question about something they have experienced, generate data, evaluate the data, and use the data to answer the question they have asked. Students question, experiment, search, theorize, and apply to life. (See also **QuESTA.**)

Seed — In a plant, the part that has the function of creating a new generation. Seeds have three parts: the **embryo,** the **endosperm,** and the **seed coat.** The embryo grows into a new plant. The endosperm provides nutrients to the embryo. The seed coat protects the seed.

Seed coat — In a **seed,** a protective outer layer, made mostly of fiber, which protects the **embryo.**

Self-pollinate — A term meaning that a flower that has both **stamen** and **pistils** can pollinate itself. An example is a peanut flower.

Sepals — Leaf-like structures that are in a ring around the base of a **flower.** They may be green or brightly colored. They protect the bud before it blossoms into a full flower.

Spines — Leaves whose primary purpose is to protect a plant.

Stamen — In a **flower,** the male reproductive part. It consists of a thin **stalk** called a filament supporting an **anther.**

Stem — In a plant, the part that transports water, minerals, sugar, and other materials throughout the plant. Stems also support the **leaves** and other plant parts, like the **flowers** and **fruit.**

Stigma — In a **flower,** the top part of the female reproductive organs. It receives the pollen.

Stoma (plural **stomata**) — An opening found in the **leaf** of a plant, that opens and closes to let gases, like carbon dioxide and oxygen, move in and out of the leaf.

Style — In a **flower,** the middle part of the female reproductive organs. It connects the **stigma** and the **ovary.**

Sustainability — The ability to provide for the needs of the present without compromising the ability of future generations to meet their own needs. For example, the ability of an ecosystem to maintain ecological processes and functions, biological diversity, and productivity over time.

Sustainable agriculture — Farming methods that provide a secure living for farm families; maintain the natural environment and resources; and support the rural community, from farm workers and consumers to the animals raised for food. (Contrast with **agribusiness.**)

Synthesis — Putting together. As in **"photosynthesis,"** putting together with light.

Technology — Mechanisms for accomplishing tasks or distributing messages and the application of knowledge to meet the goals and help provide goods and services desired by people.

Transporting — Carrying, moving, or conveying from one place to another. Apples are transported from a farm to stores or the green market in many different ways.

Tuber — An underground stem that stores food for the plant.

Variable — In an experiment, the condition or factor that is being tested. It is what will be different between the **control group** and the **experimental group.** For example, in an experiment to determine what would happen to a plant that does not get sunlight, the variable would be the amount of light the plants get.

Work — Activity that we are able to perform due to the release of stored energy in our bodies.

Xylem — A tissue in vascular plants that transports water and nutrients from the **roots** to places throughout the plant.